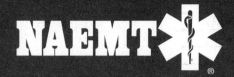

In Cooperation With

ACS / AMERICAN COLLEGE OF SURGEONS

THE COMMITTEE

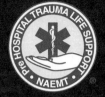

PHTLS

Prehospital Trauma Life Support

TENTH EDITION

Course Manual

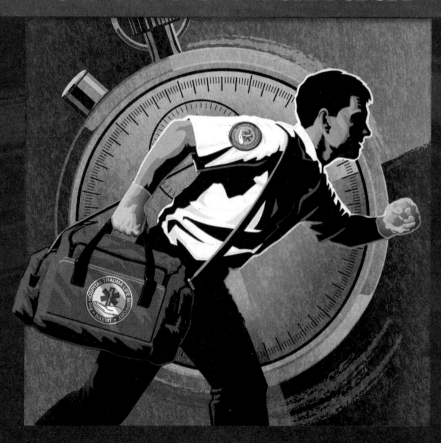

Endorsed By

east
Eastern Association for the
Surgery of Trauma

Special Operations
Medical Association

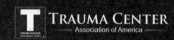

TRAUMA CENTER
Association of America

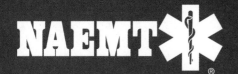
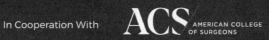 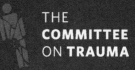

In Cooperation With

PHTLS

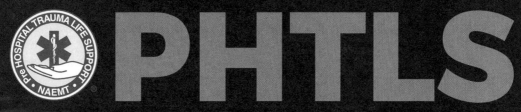

Prehospital Trauma Life Support

TENTH EDITION

Course Manual

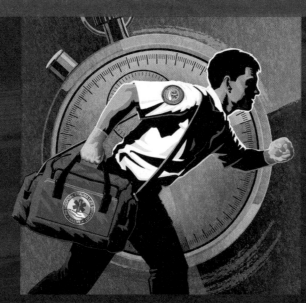

Endorsed By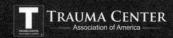

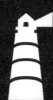

World Headquarters
Jones & Bartlett Learning
25 Mall Road
Burlington, MA 01803
978-443-5000
info@jblearning.com
www.jblearning.com
www.psglearning.com

Jones & Bartlett Learning books and products are available through most bookstores and online booksellers. To contact Jones & Bartlett Learning Public Safety Group directly, call 800-832-0034, fax 978-443-8000, or visit our website, www.psglearning.com.

Substantial discounts on bulk quantities of Jones & Bartlett Learning publications are available to corporations, professional associations, and other qualified organizations. For details and specific discount information, contact the special sales department at Jones & Bartlett Learning via the above contact information or send an email to specialsales@jblearning.com.

Copyright © 2024 by the National Association of Emergency Medical Technicians

All rights reserved. No part of the material protected by this copyright may be reproduced or utilized in any form, electronic or mechanical, including photocopying, recording, or by any information storage and retrieval system, without written permission from the copyright owner.

The content, statements, views, and opinions herein are the sole expression of the respective authors and not that of Jones & Bartlett Learning, LLC. Reference herein to any specific commercial product, process, or service by trade name, trademark, manufacturer, or otherwise does not constitute or imply its endorsement or recommendation by Jones & Bartlett Learning, LLC and such reference shall not be used for advertising or product endorsement purposes. All trademarks displayed are the trademarks of the parties noted herein. *Prehospital Trauma Life Support Course Manual, Tenth Edition* is an independent publication and has not been authorized, sponsored, or otherwise approved by the owners of the trademarks or service marks referenced in this product.

There may be images in this book that feature models; these models do not necessarily endorse, represent, or participate in the activities represented in the images. Any screenshots in this product are for educational and instructive purposes only. Any individuals and scenarios featured in the case studies throughout this product may be real or fictitious but are used for instructional purposes only.

The procedures and protocols in this book are based on the most current recommendations of responsible medical sources. The National Association of Emergency Medical Technicians (NAEMT) and the publisher, however, make no guarantee as to, and assume no responsibility for, the correctness, sufficiency, or completeness of such information or recommendations. Other or additional safety measures may be required under particular circumstances.

This textbook is intended solely as a guide to the appropriate procedures to be employed when rendering emergency care to the sick and injured. It is not intended as a statement of the standards of care required in any particular situation, because circumstances and the patient's physical condition can vary widely from one emergency to another. Nor is it intended that this textbook shall in any way advise emergency personnel concerning legal authority to perform the activities or procedures discussed. Such local determination should be made only with the aid of legal counsel.

26475-4

Production Credits

Vice President, Product Management: Marisa R. Urbano
Vice President, Content Strategy and Implementation: Christine Emerton
Director, Product Management: Laura Carney
Director, Content Management: Donna Gridley
Manager, Content Strategy: Tiffany Sliter
Content Strategist: Ashley Procum
Content Coordinator: Mark Restuccia
Development Editor: Heather Ehlers
Director, Project Management and Content Services: Karen Scott
Manager, Project Management: Jackie Reynen
Program Manager: Rachel DiMaggio
Project Manager: Madelene Nieman
Senior Digital Project Specialist: Angela Dooley

Director, Marketing: Brian Rooney
Vice President, International Sales, Public Safety Group: Matthew Maniscalco
Director, Sales, Public Safety Group: Brian Hendrickson
Content Services Manager: Colleen Lamy
Product Fulfillment Manager: Wendy Kilborn
Composition: S4Carlisle Publishing Services
Cover and Text Design: Scott Moden
Senior Media Development Editor: Troy Liston
Rights & Permissions Manager: John Rusk
Rights Specialist: Liz Kincaid
Cover Image (Title Page): © Ralf Hiemisch/Getty Images; © National Association of Emergency Medical Technicians (NAEMT)
Printing and Binding: Lakeside Book Company

Library of Congress Cataloging-in-Publication Data
Library of Congress Cataloging-in-Publication Data unavailable at time of printing.

LCCN: 2023001704

6048

Printed in the United States of America
27 26 25 24 23   10 9 8 7 6 5 4 3 2 1

Brief Contents

Table of Contents

Preface

The National Association of Emergency Medical Technicians (NAEMT) and the NAEMT Prehospital Trauma (PHT) committee, along with our partners at Jones & Bartlett Learning Public Safety Group, are pleased to present *PHTLS: Prehospital Trauma Life Support Course Manual* to accompany the 10th edition of the PHTLS course and textbook.

In revising the PHTLS course, the PHTLS course author team carefully considered feedback from PHTLS faculty and students around the world. The course schedule (and the chapters of this course manual) now follow the primary survey, with lessons on X, A, B, C, D, and E, as indicated by faculty as an intuitive approach to teaching. Course lessons continue to follow a case-based approach that encourages critical thinking and student engagement. These cases are reflected in the course manual.

The *PHTLS Course Manual* was created to enhance the course experience for all participants. The 10th edition PHTLS textbook continues as the gold-standard reference book, containing the full spectrum of medical science for prehospital trauma care.

This 10th edition course manual presents content specific to the course lessons and case studies, and it highlights key knowledge from the course to give you, the student, a deeper understanding of the content. It includes content presented by the instructor, as well as direction on where to find further information in the PHTLS textbook, so that you can access this information after the course.

The PHT committee designed the 10th edition of the PHTLS course to utilize both the textbook and the course manual to ensure that students receive the maximum educational benefits before, during, and after the 16 hours of classroom content.

—The PHTLS course author team

Acknowledgments

© Ralf Hiemisch/Getty Images

PHTLS Course Author Team

Kevin T. Collopy, MHL, FP-C, NRP, CMTE
Clinical Outcomes and Compliance
   Manager
Novant Health AirLink/VitaLink
Wilmington, North Carolina

Anthony Harbour, BSN, MEd, RN, NRP
Member, PHT Committee
Acute Care/EMS Educator, Center for
   Trauma and Critical Care Education
Virginia Commonwealth University,
   School of Medicine
Richmond, Virginia
Director, Southern Virginia EMS
Roanoke, Virginia
Goochland County Department of
   Fire-Rescue and Emergency Services
Goochland, Virginia

**Jim McKendry, BSc, MEM, ACP
(Retired)**
Member, PHT Committee
Winnipeg, Manitoba, Canada

John C. Phelps II, DBA, ACHE, NRP
NAEMT Texas State Education
   Coordinator
Healthcare Education and Business
   Consultant
San Antonio, Texas

Joanne Piccininni, MBA, NRP, MICP
Member, PHT Committee
Program Director, Assistant Professor
Bergen Community College Paramedic
   Science Program
Lyndhurst, New Jersey

Jean-Cyrille Pitteloud, MD
At-Large Member, PHT Committee
Head of Anesthesiology, HJBE Hospital
Bern County, Switzerland
Chair of the Board for Acute Care
   Anesthesia, the Swiss Society of
   Anesthesiology (SGAR)
Sion, Switzerland

Brian Simonson, MBA, NRP, CHEC
Member, PHT Committee
SERAC Trauma Coordinator
Novant New Hanover Regional Medical
   Center
Wilmington, North Carolina

NAEMT Editorial Director

Nancy Hoffmann, MSW
Senior Director of Education,
   Publishing
National Association of Emergency
   Medical Technicians

PHTLS Course Manual Editor

Kristen Lovell
National Association of Emergency
   Medical Technicians

PHTLS Course Contributors

Michael Aguilar
Justin Arnone
Debra L. Bell
Victoria Gallaher
John-David Graziano
Kris Manzano
Richard Maricle
Amy Marsh
Robert Moya
Jonathan Willoughby

NAEMT Prehospital Trauma (PHT) Committee

Dennis W. Rowe, EMT-P
Chair, PHT Committee
Director of Government and Industry
   Relations
Priority Ambulance
Knoxville, Tennessee

PHTLS Medical Director

Warren Dorlac, MD, FACS
Medical Director, PHT Committee
Colonel (Retired), USAF, MC, FS
Medical Director, Trauma and Acute
   Care Surgery
Medical Center of the Rockies
University of Colorado Health
Loveland, Colorado

PHTLS Associate Medical Director

Margaret M. Morgan, MD, FACS
Associate Medical Director, PHT
   Committee
CAPT, MC (FS/FMF), USNR
Medical Director, Perioperative
   Services
UC Health Memorial
Colorado Springs, Colorado

PHTLS Medical Editor

Andrew N. Pollak, MD
PHTLS Medical Editor
The James Lawrence Kernan Professor
   and Chairman
Department of Orthopaedics
University of Maryland School of Medicine
Chief Clinical Officer
University of Maryland Medical System
Medical Director
Baltimore County Fire Department
Special Deputy U.S. Marshal
Baltimore, Maryland

PHTLS Tactical Medical Director

**Alexander L. Eastman, MD, MPH,
FACS, FAEMS**
Tactical Medical Director, PHT Committee
Senior Medical Officer—Operations
Medical Operations/Office of the Chief
   Medical Officer
Countering Weapons of Mass
   Destruction Office
U.S. Department of Homeland Security
Washington, District of Columbia

PHT Committee Members

Frank Butler, MD
Military Medical Advisor, PHT
   Committee
CAPT, MC, USN (Retired)
Tactical Combat Casualty Care
   Consultant to the Joint Trauma System
Pensacola, Florida

Jean-Cyrille Pitteloud, MD
At-Large Member, PHT Committee
Head of Anesthesiology, HJBE Hospital
Bern County, Switzerland
Chair of the Board for Acute Care
    Anesthesia of the Swiss Society of
    Anesthesiology (SGAR)
Sion, Switzerland

Anthony Harbour, BSN, MEd, RN, NRP
Member, PHT Committee
Acute Care/EMS Educator, Center for
    Trauma and Critical Care Education
Virginia Commonwealth University,
    School of Medicine
Richmond, Virginia
Director, Southern Virginia EMS
Roanoke, Virginia
Goochland County Department of Fire-
    Rescue and Emergency Services
Goochland, Virginia

**Jim McKendry, BSc, MEM, ACP
(Retired)**
Member, PHT Committee
Winnipeg, Manitoba, Canada

Joanne Piccininni, MBA, NRP, MICP
Member, PHT Committee
Program Director, Assistant Professor
Bergen Community College Paramedic
    Science Program
Lyndhurst, New Jersey

Brian Simonson, MBA, NRP, CHEC
Member, PHT Committee
SERAC Trauma Coordinator
Novant New Hanover Regional Medical
    Center
Wilmington, North Carolina

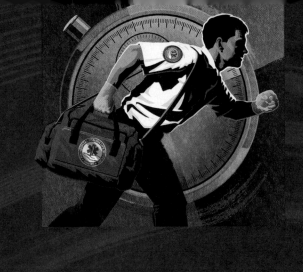

CHAPTER 1

Introduction and Overview of PHTLS

LESSON OBJECTIVES

- Identify the PHTLS course components and expectations.
- Recognize the magnitude of the human and financial impact of traumatic injury.
- Explain PHTLS goals and philosophy.
- Apply the XABCDE approach to patient assessment.
- Differentiate between principles and preferences.
- List the three phases of trauma care.
- Relate the importance of the "Golden Hour" or "Golden Period."

Introduction

Welcome to *Prehospital Trauma Life Support (PHTLS)*! This 10th edition of the PHTLS course was created by a team of subject matter experts, including instructors, emergency medical services (EMS) practitioners, and physicians from around the world. They have worked to create a course based on the latest medical evidence that represents current best practices for prehospital care of the trauma patient.

This course manual is a companion to the course and a supplement to the PHTLS text. As the PHTLS text acknowledges, this course ultimately benefits the person who needs our help—the patient. At the end of each run, we should feel that the patient received nothing short of our very best.

The overarching objectives for the PHTLS course are that at completion, you should be able to:

- Demonstrate the assessment of a trauma patient.
- Recognize priorities and establish a prehospital management plan for a patient experiencing traumatic injuries.
- Identify techniques to stop exsanguinating hemorrhage, establish a patent airway, and restore circulation in a patient with traumatic injuries.
- Describe the pathophysiology and management of traumatic brain and spinal cord injuries.

- Identify priorities of care when responding to multiple trauma patients.
- Recognize relevant trauma assessment, management, and transport considerations for geriatric, pediatric, and other special populations.
- Demonstrate the management and appropriate clinical interventions for a multisystem trauma patient.

Societal Impacts of Trauma

Injuries and deaths from trauma have a direct impact not only on those involved, but also on society as a whole. Each year, approximately 4.4 million people in the world die as a result of injury, accounting for nearly 8% of all deaths. The combined total of deaths caused by diseases such as tuberculosis, malaria, and HIV/AIDS amounts to only a little more than half the number of deaths that result from injury. For further perspective, approximately 3 million people died during the first (and hopefully deadliest) year of the COVID-19 pandemic. Although it is not difficult to see that trauma is a problem of pandemic proportions that occurs each and every year, understanding the cause of traumatic injury and the most effective means of treating it remains complicated, despite the abundance of data available on the subject.

Main Causes of Death Due to Trauma

Drowning and motor vehicle collisions (MVCs) are substantial causes of death in early life; drowning deaths decrease greatly after age 25, whereas MVCs continue to increase until surpassed by falls at age 65. In fact, MVCs and falls are the only causes of death resulting from trauma expected to increase globally by 2030, due to an increase in the number of vehicles and related infrastructure and an aging population, respectively.

Examining fall- and MVC-related deaths illustrates some of the complications that are found in addressing unintentional injury and trauma on a universal scale. The number-one cause of nonfatal injuries in the United States in 2019 was unintentional falls. Unintentional injury is the leading cause of death between the ages of 1 and 45 years (**Figure 1-1**), and it results in 14,000 deaths each day worldwide (**Figure 1-2**).

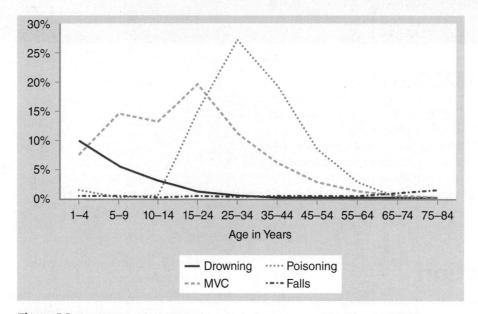

Figure 1-1 Percentage of all deaths by selected cause—ages 1 to 85 years, 2019.

Data from the National Center for Injury Prevention and Control: WISQARS. 10 leading causes of death, United States, 2019, all races, both sexes. Centers for Disease Control and Prevention. https://wisqars.cdc.gov/fatal-leading

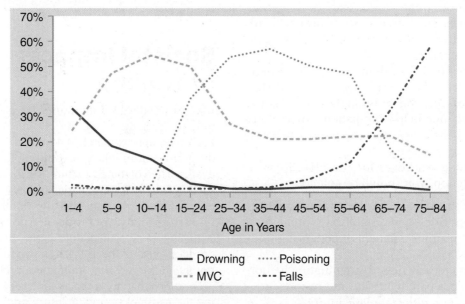

Figure 1-2 Percentage of unintentional injury deaths by selected cause—ages 1 to 85 years, 2019.

Data from the National Center for Injury Prevention and Control: WISQARS. 10 leading causes of death, United States, 2019, all races, both sexes. Centers for Disease Control and Prevention. https://wisqars.cdc.gov/fatal-leading

Although not considered a traumatic cause of death, poisoning is growing as a leading cause of death secondary to unintentional injury—a trend likely to continue into the future if the opioid epidemic persists.

> **CRITICAL THINKING QUESTION**
>
> On an individual level, think of the devastating impact an injury can have on quality of life. Can you think of some examples you have witnessed? Could those injuries have been prevented?

> **FOR MORE INFORMATION**
>
> *Refer to the "Philosophy of PHTLS" section of Chapter 1: PHTLS: Past, Present, and Future in the PHTLS 10th edition main text.*

Financial Impacts of Trauma

Although the loss of life due to trauma is staggering, so, too, is the financial burden of caring for the patients who survive. Billions of dollars are spent on the management of trauma patients, not including the dollars lost in wages, insurance administration costs, property damage, and employer costs.

The National Safety Council estimated that the economic impact in 2019 from both fatal and non-fatal trauma was approximately $1.1 trillion in the United States. Saving an individual life by identifying life-threatening hemorrhage, and transporting patients expeditiously to a trauma center for resuscitation and hemorrhage control, can save society $1.2 million per patient in lifetime wage and productivity losses. Per-patient costs associated with cancer and heart disease are much lower. The National Safety Council's (NSC's) Injury Facts webpage is a great resource to learn more about the societal costs of trauma (https://injuryfacts.nsc.org/all-injuries/costs/societal-costs/).

> **QUICK TIP**
>
> By using the knowledge and skills taught in PHTLS, you can reduce the costs of trauma. For example, protecting a patient's fractured cervical spine properly may make the difference between quadriplegia and a healthy life with unrestricted activity.

> **CRITICAL THINKING QUESTION**
>
> What is one change you can make in your daily practice that can help reduce trauma costs in your community?

> **FOR MORE INFORMATION**
>
> *Refer to the "Epidemiology and Financial Burden" section of Chapter 1: PHTLS: Past, Present, and Future in the PHTLS 10th edition main text.*

Goals of PHTLS

The goals of PHTLS are simple and clear:

- Reduce mortality and injury from trauma.
- Provide prehospital care practitioners with knowledge and skills.
- Provide appropriate care to trauma patients.

To help achieve these goals, you will apply your critical thinking skills in the field. Critical thinking in medicine is a process in which the healthcare practitioner assesses the situation, the patient, and the resources available and uses the information to decide on and provide the best care for the patient (**Figure 1-3**). The critical thinking process requires you to:

- Develop a plan of action.
- Initiate the plan.
- Reassess the plan as care for the patient moves forward.
- Adjust the plan as the patient's condition or circumstances change.

> **Components of Critical Thinking in Emergency Medical Care**
>
> 1. Assess the situation.
> 2. Assess the patient.
> 3. Assess the available resources.
> 4. Analyze the possible solutions.
> 5. Select the best answer to manage the situation and patient.
> 6. Develop the plan of action.
> 7. Initiate the plan of action.
> 8. Reassess the response of the patient to the plan of action.
> 9. Make any needed adjustments or changes to the plan of action.
> 10. Continue with steps 8 and 9 until this phase of care is completed.

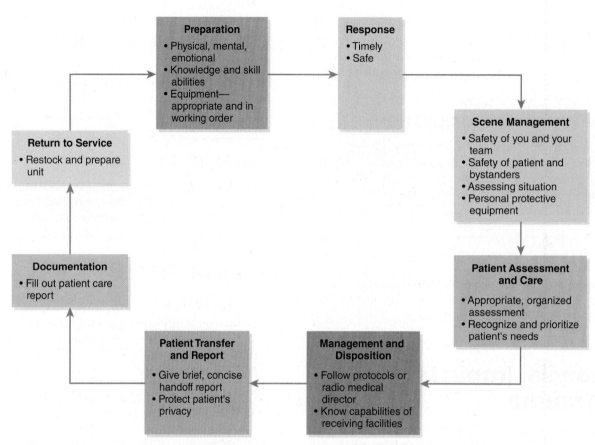

Figure 1-3 Prehospital care practitioners follow an important sequence of procedures for each emergency call.
© Jones & Bartlett Learning

> **FOR MORE INFORMATION**
>
> *Refer to the "Critical Thinking" section of Chapter 2: Golden Principles, Preferences, and Critical Thinking in the PHTLS 10th edition main text.*

Philosophy of PHTLS

PHTLS does not advocate for or train prehospital care practitioners to memorize a "one-size-fits-all" approach. Rather, the PHTLS philosophy holds that prehospital care practitioners must possess and apply critical thinking skills to rapidly make and carry out decisions that will enhance the survival of trauma patients. Each prehospital care practitioner–patient contact presents a unique set of circumstances. If the prehospital care practitioner understands the basis of medical care and the specific needs of the individual patient given the circumstances at hand, then precise patient care decisions can be made that ensure the greatest chance of survival for that patient.

The overarching tenets of PHTLS are that prehospital care practitioners:

- Must have a good foundation of knowledge
- Must be critical thinkers
- Must have appropriate technical skills to deliver excellent patient care, even in less-than-optimal circumstances

Interventions: What Do We Do?

Appropriate interventions in prehospital trauma care are based on the assessment of each patient. Often, knowing when *not* to do something is more important than knowing when to do it. Although this course focuses on trauma interventions, PHTLS neither recommends nor prohibits specific actions for the prehospital care practitioner. Appropriate skills and interventions are determined by local protocols and by critical cost-benefit evaluation.

Patient Care Delivery: How Do We Do It?

Patient care delivery focuses on delivering the trauma patient to the right facility, utilizing the right mode of transport, in the right amount of time, as safely as possible.

FOR MORE INFORMATION

Refer to the "Philosophy of PHTLS" section of Chapter 1: PHTLS: Past, Present, and Future and the "Research" section of Chapter 2: Golden Principles, Preferences, and Critical Thinking in the PHTLS 10th edition main text.

Team Approach

PHTLS stresses using a team approach for patient care that includes a variety of players ranging in knowledge and skills (**Figure 1-4**). The team approach goes beyond just patient care—it also includes research, data collection, and prevention programs that can help decrease the number of traumatic events each year. In addition to EMS personnel, the players on the trauma prevention, assessment, and care team include:

- Citizens
- Dispatchers
- Law enforcement
- Fire personnel
- Highway safety experts
- Hospital personnel
- Rehabilitation services
- Primary care practitioners

Trauma is a global problem, and prevention is a vital part of our job. Working together provides trauma patients with the highest chance of survival.

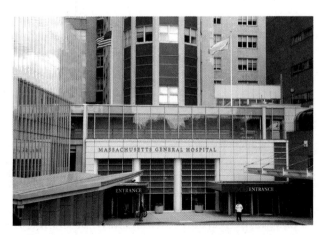

Figure 1-4 Working together—both in the field and in the hospital—provides trauma patients with the highest chance of survival.
© Elise Amendola/AP Photo

Assessment and Treatment of Trauma Patients

PHTLS provides an understanding of anatomy and physiology, the pathophysiology of trauma, and the assessment and care of the trauma patient. The standard trauma survey uses the XABCDE approach to patient

XABCDE

PHTLS uses XABCDE in the primary survey to recognize the immediate and potentially irreversible threat posed by exsanguinating extremity or junctional hemorrhage. The "X" placed before the traditional "ABCDE" describes the need to address exsanguinating hemorrhage immediately after establishing scene safety and before addressing airway. Severe exsanguinating hemorrhage, particularly arterial bleeding, has the potential to lead to the loss of total or near total blood volume in a relatively short period of time. Depending on the pace of the bleeding, that time can be just a few minutes. Thus, even prior to airway stabilization, controlling severe bleeding from a limb or other compressible external site takes precedence. This is followed by managing airway threats, ensuring adequate breathing, assessing circulatory status, determining the extent of disability, and exposing the body to allow a thorough evaluation.

- **X**—eXsanguinating hemorrhage
- **A**—Airway
- **B**—Breathing
- **C**—Circulation
- **D**—Disability
- **E**—Expose/Environment

QUICK TIP

MARCH and the CABCDE approach may still be used in some areas or organizations. MARCH stands for Massive bleeding, Airway, Respirations, Circulation, Head injury/Hypothermia. CABCDE stands for Catastrophic hemorrhage control, Airway, Breathing, Circulation, Disability, Expose/Environment. Although different organizations may use these acronyms, they all reflect the same priorities of patient assessment.

assessment. Patients who are bleeding or breathing inadequately do not have much time before their condition results in disability or becomes fatal.

PHTLS: Past, Present, Future

Past

A personal experience brought about the changes in emergency care that resulted in the Advanced Trauma Life Support (ATLS) course and, eventually, the PHTLS program. ATLS started in 1978, two years after a private plane crash in a rural area of Nebraska, where an orthopedic surgeon's wife was killed and his children were critically injured. The surgeon recognized the lack of a trauma care delivery system to treat acutely injured patients in rural settings. He and his colleagues decided that rural physicians needed to be trained in a systematic manner on treating trauma patients. They chose to use a format similar to Advanced Cardiovascular Life Support (ACLS) and called it Advanced Trauma Life Support. The ATLS course, developed and revised by the American College of Surgeons Committee on Trauma (ACS COT), is the basis of PHTLS.

Present

The first chairman of the ATLS ad hoc committee for the American College of Surgeons (ACS) and Chairman of the Prehospital Care Subcommittee on Trauma for the American College of Surgeons, Dr. Norman E. McSwain Jr., FACS, knew that ATLS would have a profound effect on the outcomes of trauma patients (**Figure 1-5**). Moreover, he had a strong sense that an even greater effect could come from bringing this type of critical training to prehospital care practitioners.

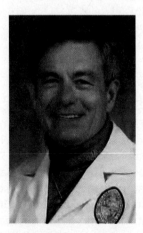

Figure 1-5 Dr. Norman E. McSwain Jr., helped transform prehospital trauma care.
Courtesy Norman McSwain, MD, FACS, NREMT-P.

Dr. McSwain, a founding member of the board of directors of the National Association of Emergency Medical Technicians (NAEMT), put together the draft curriculum of what would become PHTLS.

> **Strong Partnerships Make Good Practitioners**
>
> Throughout the growth of PHTLS, medical oversight has been provided through the ACS COT. For over 30 years, the partnership between the ACS and NAEMT has ensured that PHTLS course participants receive the opportunity to give trauma patients their best chance at survival.

Vision for the Future

The PHTLS program brings together the work of practitioners and researchers around the globe to determine standards of trauma care for the new millennium. PHTLS is currently taught in over 70 countries worldwide. (For a current list of countries, see https://www.naemt.org/education/naemt-education-worldwide/.)

As prehospital trauma care evolves and improves, so, too, must the PHTLS program. We are dedicated to ongoing evaluation of the program to identify and implement improvements wherever needed. We will pursue new methods and technology for delivering PHTLS to enhance the clinical and service quality of the program.

> FOR MORE INFORMATION
>
> *Refer to the "PHTLS—Past, Present, Future" section of Chapter 1: PHTLS: Past, Present, and Future in the PHTLS 10th edition main text.*

Principles and Preferences

The science of medicine provides the principles of medical care. Simply stated, *principles* define the duties required of the prehospital care practitioner in optimizing patient survival and outcome. How these principles are implemented to most efficiently manage the patient depends on the *preferences*, which describe how a system and its individual practitioners choose to apply scientific principles to the care of patients. Preferences could change depending on the situation, the number of patients and the severity of their injuries, the practitioner's knowledge and skills, and available resources.

Let us take airway management, for example:

- The *principle* is that air, containing oxygen, must be moved through an open airway into the alveoli of the lungs to facilitate oxygen–carbon dioxide exchange with red blood cells (RBCs) so they may deliver oxygen to other tissues.
- The *preference* is how airway management is implemented in a particular patient. In some cases, patients will manage their own airway; in other cases, the prehospital care practitioner will have to decide which adjunct is best to facilitate airway management. The practitioner will determine the best method to ensure that the air passages are open to get oxygen into the lungs and, secondarily, to get carbon dioxide out.

Principles Versus Preferences

- A *principle* is the basis for maximizing a patient's chance of survival.
- A *preference* is how the principle is implemented.

CRITICAL THINKING QUESTION

Can you think of a time when you had to employ a principle over your own preference?

The foundation of PHTLS is to teach prehospital care practitioners to make appropriate decisions for patient care based on knowledge, not protocol. The goal of patient care is to achieve the principle. How this is achieved (i.e., the decision made by the practitioner to manage the patient) is the preference based on the situation, patient condition, fund of knowledge and skill, local protocols, and equipment available at the time.

FOR MORE INFORMATION

Refer to the "Principles and Preferences" section of PHTLS Chapter 2: Golden Principles, Preferences, and Critical Thinking in the PHTLS 10th edition main text.

The Phases of Trauma Care

Traumatic incidents fall into two categories: *intentional* and *unintentional*. Intentional injury results from an act carried out on purpose with the goal of harming, injuring, or killing. Traumatic injury that occurs as an unintended or accidental consequence is considered unintentional.

Trauma care is divided into three phases:

1. Pre-event
2. Event
3. Post-event

Actions can be taken to minimize the impact of traumatic injury during any of these three phases. You have critical responsibilities during each phase.

Pre-event Phase

The pre-event phase involves the circumstances leading up to an injury. Efforts are primarily focused on injury prevention. For example, approximately 85% of Americans owned a smartphone in 2021, compared to 35% in 2011. This growth has been associated with a progressive increase in the number of deaths due to distracted driving. The Centers for Disease Control and Prevention estimates that distracted driving results in approximately 3,000 deaths per year, with younger drivers at disproportionately higher risk. Prevention efforts have taken place to curb this rising trend, such as legal enforcement aimed specifically at preventing traffic accidents and public awareness campaigns such as "It Can Wait" and "U Drive. U Text. U Pay." To achieve maximum effect, strategies in the pre-event phase should focus on the most significant contributors to mortality and morbidity.

Promoting programs that raise awareness among populations at risk for falling is another area of significant public health effort. Prehospital care practitioners are in a unique position to play a role in fall prevention. With one of the leading risk factors for a fall resulting in injury or death among older adults being a previous fall incident, it is possible that local EMS personnel are encountering at-risk individuals during calls for lift assistance or minor injury. EMS practitioners are also one of the few members of the healthcare team who interact with patients in their own homes, which allows EMS personnel to observe patients' living conditions and point out tripping hazards like loose rugs, inadequate lighting, and other fall-related risks. These calls present an important opportunity for local public safety departments to collaborate with other healthcare practitioners and organizations to develop an evidence-based fall prevention program in the community. See NAEMT's Injury and Illness Prevention webpage for resources: https://naemt.org/initiatives/prevention/.

Prepare for the Unpreventable

As a prehospital care practitioner, you need to prepare for events that are not preventable by:

- Maintaining your education on the most current evidence-based medical practices
- Updating your medical knowledge (much like you update your handheld devices)
- Reviewing new and current equipment on your response unit at the beginning of your shift and in trainings
- Understanding individual responsibilities and expectations of shift and patient care duties
- Understanding how to make the best use of your environment and your resources (e.g., roads, hospitals)

Event Phase

The event phase is the moment of the actual trauma. Actions taken during this phase are aimed at minimizing injury resulting from the trauma. The use of safety equipment has a major influence on the severity of injury caused by the traumatic event; examples include:

- Motor vehicle safety restraint systems
- Air bags
- Motorcycle helmets
- Child safety seats

Fix It and Click It

Many trauma centers, law enforcement organizations, and EMS and fire systems conduct programs to educate parents on the correct installation and use of child safety seats. When correctly installed and properly used, child safety seats offer infants and children the best protection during the event phase of trauma care.

Whether driving a personal vehicle or an emergency vehicle, you need to protect yourself and teach by example. You are responsible for yourself, your partner, and the patients under your care while in your ambulance or vehicle. It is your responsibility to prevent injury with safe and attentive driving. Always use the personal protective devices available, such as vehicle restraints, in the driving compartment and in the passenger or patient care compartment.

Post-event Phase

The post-event phase deals with the outcome of the traumatic event. The worst possible outcome is death of

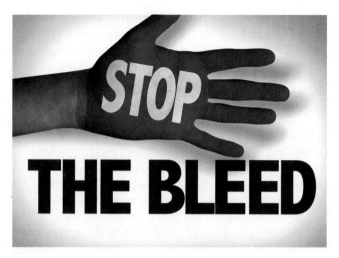

Figure 1-6 Immediate deaths can be prevented by injury prevention strategies and public education programs. Early deaths can be prevented through timely, appropriate prehospital care to reduce mortality and morbidity. Late deaths can be prevented only through prompt transport to a hospital appropriately staffed for trauma care.
© Gustavo Frazao/Shutterstock

the patient. Many of these deaths can be prevented and outcomes in trauma patients improved by exemplary prehospital care and hospital care (**Figure 1-6**), including:

- Early and aggressive management of shock
- Aggressive hemorrhage control
- Damage control resuscitation in the hospital

One of your most important responsibilities as a prehospital care practitioner is to spend as little time on the scene as possible and expedite your field care and transport of the patient. Studies show that the time from injury to arrival at the appropriate trauma center is critical to survival.

Golden Period: How Much Time Does a Patient Have?

In the late 1960s, R. Adams Cowley, MD, conceived the idea of a crucial time period during which definitive patient care should begin for a critically injured trauma patient; this came to be known as the "Golden Hour." The "hour" was intended to be figurative and not a literal description of a period of time. A patient with a penetrating wound to the heart may have only a few minutes to reach definitive care before shock becomes irreversible, but a patient with slow, ongoing internal hemorrhage from an isolated fracture may have several hours or longer to reach definitive care and resuscitation.

Because the Golden Hour is not a strict 60-minute time frame and varies from patient to patient based on the injuries, we often use the term *Golden Period*. The ACS COT has used this concept to emphasize the importance of transporting trauma patients to facilities where expert trauma care is available in a timely manner.

Golden Period: Critical Timing!

Some patients have less than an hour in which to receive care, whereas others have more time. In many urban prehospital systems in the United States, the average time between activation of EMS and arrival to the scene is 8 to 9 minutes, not including the time between injury and the call to the public safety answering point. A typical transport time to the receiving facility is another 8 to 9 minutes. If the prehospital care practitioners spend only 10 minutes on the scene, over 30 minutes of time will have already passed by the time a patient arrives at the receiving facility. Every additional minute spent on scene is additional time that the patient is bleeding, and valuable time is ticking away from the Golden Period.

One of the most important responsibilities of a prehospital care practitioner is to expedite the field care and transport of the patient. In the 2000s, prehospital scene times have decreased by allowing all practitioners (fire, police, and EMS) to work as a cohesive team by using a standard methodology across emergency services. As a result, patient survival has increased.

A second responsibility is transporting the patient to an appropriate facility. A factor that is extremely critical to a compromised patient's survival is the length of time that elapses between the incident and the provision of definitive care. Trauma center designations are developed at local or state levels, and the regulations for what resources must be available for each category of trauma center (level I, level II, level III, etc.) vary from state to state. The ACS evaluates trauma centers to verify the presence of resources listed in the ACS

Golden Period Goals

1. **Gain access** to the patient.
2. **Identify and treat** life-threatening injuries.
3. **Minimize** on-scene time through rapid assessment, rapid patient packaging, and limiting on-scene treatments to only those that reverse immediately life-threatening conditions.
4. **Transport** the patient to the closest appropriate facility by the most expeditious mode of transport.

---

document, *Resources for Optimal Care of the Injured Patient*. A description of the different levels of trauma centers can be found on the Brain Trauma Foundation's website: https://braintrauma.org/news/article/trauma-center-designations.

FOR MORE INFORMATION

Refer to "The Phases of Trauma Care" section of Chapter 1: PHTLS: Past, Present, and Future in the PHTLS 10th edition main text.

Communication and Documentation

Communication about a trauma patient with the receiving hospital involves three components:

1. Prearrival warning
2. Verbal report upon arrival
3. Written documentation of the encounter in the patient care report (PCR)

Care of the trauma patient is a team effort. The response to a critical trauma patient begins with the prehospital care practitioner and continues in the hospital. Delivering information from the prehospital setting to the receiving hospital allows for notification and mobilization of appropriate hospital resources to ensure an optimal reception of the patient.

Write It Down

Effective documentation, as provided in the PCR, fulfills several key functions:

- Maintains continuity of high-quality patient care
- Documents the assessment and management of the patient in the field for legal purposes
- Supports and continues trauma research
- Supports trauma system funding

Reflect, Research, and Adapt

- We must critically examine how and why we do everything.
- Science is always evolving, helping us to verify or refute our approach to trauma care.
- We must be able to adapt to changes.

SUMMARY

- The overarching tenets of Prehospital Trauma Life Support (PHTLS) are that prehospital care practitioners must have a good foundation of knowledge, must be critical thinkers, and must have appropriate technical skills to deliver excellent patient care, even in less-than-optimal circumstances.

- Worldwide, injury is a leading cause of death and disability, impacting not only the people directly involved, but also, given the magnitude of its financial ramifications, society as a whole.

- PHTLS uses XABCDE in the primary survey to recognize the immediate and potentially irreversible threat posed by exsanguinating extremity or junctional hemorrhage, stressing the need to address exsanguinating hemorrhage immediately after establishing scene safety and before addressing airway.

- Principles (or the *science* of medicine) define the duties required of the prehospital care practitioner

in optimizing patient survival and outcome. Preferences (or the *art* of medicine) are the methods of achieving the principle.

- Critical thinking in medicine is a process in which the healthcare practitioner assesses the situation, the patient, and the resources. This information is rapidly analyzed and combined to provide the best care possible to the patient.

- Improving outcomes from trauma can be considered in three phases: pre-event, event, and post-event. Actions can be taken to minimize the impact of traumatic injury during any of the three phases of trauma care. The prehospital care practitioner has critical responsibilities during each phase.

- The concept of a Golden Hour or Golden Period guides prehospital care. Research has shown that prompt transport to definitive care is key to improving patient outcomes.

STUDY QUESTIONS

1. Which of the following requires you to develop a plan of action, initiate the plan, reassess the plan as care for the patient moves forward, and adjust the plan as the patient's condition or circumstances change?
   A. Principles of PHTLS
   B. The Golden Period
   C. The XABCDE assessment
   D. Critical thinking process

2. When using the XABCDE assessment, which of the following takes precedence over all other actions?
   A. Controlling severe bleeding from a limb or other compressible site
   B. Airway stabilization and assessing circulatory status
   C. Exposing the body to allow a thorough evaluation
   D. Ensuring adequate breathing

3. Which of the following is the basis on which a patient's chance of survival is maximized?
   A. Preferences
   B. Phases
   C. Principles
   D. Transport

4. Which of the following is a goal of the Golden Period?
   A. Provide written documentation from field care to receiving hospital.
   B. Expedite the field care and transport of the patient.
   C. Use a team approach for optimal patient care.
   D. Use the XABCDE approach to patient assessment.

ANSWER KEY

Question 1: D
To help achieve the PHTLS goals, you will apply your critical thinking skills in the field. Critical thinking in medicine is a process in which the healthcare practitioner assesses the situation, the patient, and the

resources available and uses the information to decide on and provide the best care for the patient.

Question 2: A
The "X" placed before "ABCDE" in the primary survey refers to the need to address exsanguinating

hemorrhage immediately after establishing scene safety and before addressing airway. Severe exsanguinating hemorrhage, particularly arterial bleeding, has the potential to lead to loss of total or near total blood volume in a relatively short period of time.

Question 3: C
The science of medicine provides the principles of medical care. Simply stated, *principles* define the duties required of the prehospital care practitioner in optimizing patient survival and outcome.

Question 4: B
One of your most important responsibilities as a prehospital care practitioner is to spend as little time on the scene as possible and expedite your field care and transport of the patient. Studies show that the time from injury to arrival at the appropriate site for definitive care is critical to survival.

REFERENCES AND FURTHER READING

American College of Surgeons. *Resources for Optimal Care of the Injured Patient.* 6th ed. Chicago, IL: American College of Surgeons; March 2022 (effective September 2023, available currently; 2014 standards available and in place until September 2022). https://www.facs.org/quality-programs/trauma/quality/verification-review-and-consultation-program/standards/. Accessed September 14, 2021.

Brain Trauma Foundation. Trauma center designations and levels. https://braintrauma.org/news/article/trauma-center-designations/. Published January 1, 2000. Accessed September 14, 2022.

Centers for Disease Control and Prevention. Distracted driving. https://www.cdc.gov/transportationsafety/distracted_driving/index.html#problem/. Last reviewed March 2, 2021. Accessed November 11, 2021.

Centers for Disease Control and Prevention. Road traffic injuries and deaths—A global problem. https://www.cdc.gov/injury/features/global-road-safety/index.html. Last reviewed December 14, 2020. Accessed September 14, 2021.

Centers for Disease Control and Prevention. 10 leading causes of death, United States, 2019, all races, both sexes. https://wisqars.cdc.gov/fatal-leading/. Accessed November 11, 2021.

Centers for Disease Control and Prevention, National Center for Injury Prevention and Control. Fact sheet: risk factors for falls. https://www.cdc.gov/steadi/pdf/Risk_Factors_for_Falls-print.pdf. Published 2017. Accessed September 2022.

Centers for Disease Control and Prevention, National Center for Injury Prevention and Control. Preventing falls: a guide to implementing effective community-based fall prevention programs. https://www.cdc.gov/homeandrecreationalsafety/pdf/falls/fallpreventionguide-2015-a.pdf. Published 2015. Accessed September 14, 2022.

National Association of Emergency Medical Technicians. Injury and illness prevention. http://naemt.org/resources/community-education/prevention. Last updated 2018. Accessed September 13, 2022.

National Association of Emergency Medical Technicians. *PHTLS: Prehospital Trauma Life Support.* 10th ed. Burlington, MA: Public Safety Group; 2023.

National Safety Council. Injury facts: societal costs. https://injuryfacts.nsc.org/all-injuries/costs/societal-costs/. Accessed November 11, 2021.

World Health Organization. Falls. https://www.who.int/news-room/fact-sheets/detail/falls/. Published April 26, 2021. Accessed November 11, 2021.

World Health Organization. Road traffic injuries. https://www.who.int/news-room/fact-sheets/detail/road-traffic-injuries/. Published June 21, 2021. Accessed November 11, 2021.

CHAPTER 2

Trauma Assessment and X–Exsanguinating Hemorrhage

LESSON OBJECTIVES

- Describe the steps for evaluating scene safety.
- Demonstrate how to perform a trauma assessment.
- Describe methods to manage hemorrhage in the prehospital setting.
- Explain how to apply the National Field Triage Guidelines to prehospital transport decisions.
- Discuss prehospital care of traumatic cardiopulmonary arrest.
- Discuss special considerations in the assessment of trauma patients and hemorrhage management.

Introduction

Critical injuries must be definitively cared for quickly in order to optimize patient survival, and prehospital practitioners often have limited ability to manage critical injuries (e.g., internal bleeding) in the prehospital setting. The primary role of the EMS practitioner at the trauma scene is to assess and identify patient criticality and to deliver a critically injured patient to the closest medical facility able to provide definitive care. Practitioners managing critically injured patients should keep in mind the following:

- Definitive care is available at regional trauma centers.
- It is important to recognize the extent of patient injuries.
- There are limitations to scope of practice and equipment available in the prehospital setting.

Thus, to optimize patient survival, the patient should be assessed in such a way as to identify the most immediate life-threatening injury first, and transport must be initiated as soon as the need for immediate definitive care is identified. A complete assessment to identify all injuries may not be performed on scene if an immediate life threat is identified and transport initiated. (The remainder of the assessment may be performed en route.) PHTLS trauma assessment provides a systematic way to optimize patient survival.

Priorities of Care

There are a number of concerns you must be aware of when responding to a call and arriving on scene. The information gathered by the dispatch center is critical, not only for your safety, but also for that of everyone in the general area. Your assessment of the scene is a continuous event that must come with a plan of action if the need to evacuate arises.

The on-scene information-gathering process begins immediately upon arrival at the incident. Before approaching the patient, evaluate the scene by:

1. Obtaining a general impression of the situation for scene safety for responders, bystanders, and patient(s)
2. Determining the need for additional resources
3. Considering the mechanism of injury (MOI)

Once you have determined the scene is safe and you have formed an initial impression, perform the primary survey to identify life threats.

Scene Safety

The appearance of the scene influences the entire assessment. You can gather a wealth of information by simply looking, listening, and cataloging as much

CASE STUDY: DISPATCH

It is dusk during a rainstorm. You are dispatched to a highway location for a motor vehicle/cyclist collision. There is one patient: an unresponsive 24-year-old.

Questions:

- What scene safety concerns or considerations are present?
- What other patient-related information would you like to know?

Determine the Need for Additional Resources

Additional resources needed may include:

- Additional transport vehicles
- Air transport
- Fire suppression
- Extrication
- Traffic control (**Figure 2-2**)
- Hazardous materials containment
- Utilities (gas, electric)

information as possible, including the MOI, the present situation, and the overall degree of safety.

The first consideration when approaching any scene is the safety of *all* emergency responders (**Figure 2-1**). When emergency medical services (EMS) personnel become victims, they not only can no longer assist others, but also add to the number of patients. Patient care may need to wait until the scene is safe enough for you to enter without undue risk. Potential safety concerns include:

- Exposure to body fluids
- Exposure to chemical weapons used in warfare
- Fire
- Downed electrical lines
- Explosives
- Hazardous materials
- Traffic
- Floodwater
- An assailant on scene
- Adverse weather conditions

Violence

Every call has the potential to take you into an emotionally charged environment. Even a scene that appears safe has the potential to deteriorate quickly, so always be alert to subtle clues that suggest a change in the situation. The patient, family, or bystanders on the scene may not be able to perceive the situation rationally. They may think the response time was too long, be overly sensitive to words or actions, and misunderstand the "usual" approach to patient assessment.

Know Before You Go

Some EMS agencies have a policy requiring the presence of law enforcement before practitioners enter a violent or potentially violent scene. Check your local protocols.

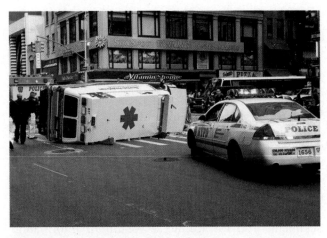

Figure 2-1 The majority of EMS personnel who are killed or injured each year were involved in motor vehicle incidents.

© Robert Brenner/PhotoEdit

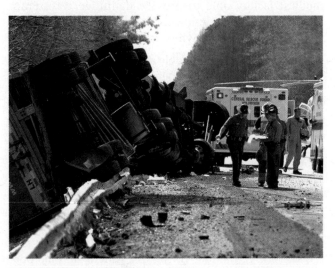

Figure 2-2 A significant number of prehospital care practitioners who are injured or killed were working at the scene of a motor vehicle collision.

© Jeff Thrower (Web Thrower)/Shutterstock

Maintaining a confident and professional manner while demonstrating respect and concern is important to gaining the patient's trust and achieving control of the scene.

It is important for you to train yourself to *observe* the scene. EMS personnel must learn to notice:

- The number and location of individuals when arriving on the scene
- The movement of bystanders into or out of the scene
- Any indicators of stress or tension
- Unexpected or unusual reactions to EMS presence

If you perceive a developing threat, *immediately prepare to leave the scene.* An assessment or a procedure may need to be completed in the ambulance. The safety of prehospital care practitioners is the first priority.

Be Aware: Look at Hands and Clothing

Watch the patient's and bystanders' hands. Look for unusual bulges in waistbands, clothing that is worn out of season, or oversized clothing that could easily hide a weapon.

Managing the Violent Scene

Partners need to discuss and agree on methods to handle a violent patient or bystander. Attempting to develop a process during the event is prone to failure. Partners can use a hands-on or hands-off approach, as well as predetermined code words and hand signals, for emergencies.

If both practitioners have all their attention focused on the patient, the scene can quickly become threatening, and early clues may be missed. In many situations, patient, family, and bystander tension and anxiety are immediately reduced when one attentive practitioner begins interacting with and assessing the patient, while the other practitioner observes the scene and communicates with the patient's family.

Mechanism of Injury

The information you gather from your scene assessment allows you and your team to forecast the injuries your patient may have suffered. The saying "a picture is worth a thousand words" holds true when dealing with a mechanism of injury (MOI). Determining the mechanism of injury can provide a clue to the amount of energy that was transferred to the patient's body and help practitioners determine what injuries were

---

Safety Strategies

There are various methods for dealing with a scene that has become dangerous, including the following:

- *Don't be there.* When responding to a known violent scene, stage at a safe location until the scene has been rendered safe by law enforcement and clearance to respond has been given.
- *Retreat.* If threats are presented when approaching the scene, tactfully retreat to the vehicle and leave the scene. Stage at a safe location and notify appropriate personnel.
- *Defuse.* If a scene becomes threatening during patient care, use verbal skills to reduce tension and aggression (while preparing to leave the scene).
- *Defend.* As a last resort, prehospital care practitioners may find it necessary to defend themselves. It is important that such efforts are to "disengage and get away." Do not attempt to chase or subdue an aggressive party. Ensure that law enforcement personnel have been notified and are en route. Again, the safety of the practitioners is the priority.

FOR MORE INFORMATION

Refer to the "Violence" section of Chapter 5: Scene Management in the PHTLS 10th edition main text.

---

sustained. Your ability to obtain this critical information and to pass that information along to the trauma center plays a profound role in patient outcome.

Primary Survey

Once you have determined that the scene is safe, you can complete a rapid patient assessment. For the trauma patient, as for other critically ill patients, assessment is the foundation on which all management and transport decisions are based. You need to develop an overall impression of a patient's status and establish baseline values for the patient's respiratory, circulatory, and neurologic systems. When life-threatening conditions are identified, you need to immediately intervene. If time and the patient's condition allow, you will

CASE STUDY: INITIAL IMPRESSION

You find one patient lying prone on the shoulder of a two-lane undivided highway. According to witnesses, the patient was riding a bicycle when he was struck from behind by a car traveling approximately 40 mph (64 kph). The cyclist landed head first on the pavement and has not moved or been moved since.

Questions:

- Remembering your priorities of care and the importance of scene safety, what are potential scene hazards?
- What methods can you use to mitigate these scene hazards?
- Are additional resources needed?
- What is your initial impression of the prone patient as you approach him? Can the patient be assessed in the prone position?

FOR MORE INFORMATION

Refer to the "Scene Assessment" and "Safety Issues" sections of Chapter 5: Scene Management in the PHTLS 10th edition main text.

conduct a secondary survey for injuries that are not life- or limb-threatening. Often this secondary survey occurs during patient transport.

Forming a general impression of the patient within the first few moments of contact is critical. Recall from Chapter 1 that the primary survey assessment is used to identify the most immediate life threats first. The primary survey must proceed rapidly and in a logical order. If you are alone, you can perform some key interventions as you identify life-threatening conditions. If more than one practitioner is present, one

Different Populations, Same Survey

The same primary survey approach is utilized regardless of the patient type. All patients, including geriatric, pediatric, or pregnant patients, are assessed in a similar fashion to ensure that all components of the assessment are covered and that no significant pathology is missed. However, additional considerations are required for specific patient populations.

may complete the primary survey while others initiate care. When several critical conditions are identified, the primary survey allows you to establish treatment priorities. In general, you should manage compressible external hemorrhage first, an airway issue is managed before a breathing problem, and so forth. Each crew member going into the scene should have a plan for their responsibilities and how they will achieve them.

When initially approaching a patient, look for severe compressible hemorrhage and check whether the patient appears to be moving air effectively, if they are awake or unresponsive, and if they are moving spontaneously. Once at the patient's side, introduce yourself to the patient and ask the patient's name. A reasonable next step is to ask the patient, "What happened to you?" If the patient appears comfortable and can answer coherently in complete sentences, you can conclude that the patient has a patent airway, sufficient respiratory function to support speech, adequate cerebral perfusion, and reasonable neurologic functioning; there are probably no immediate threats to this patient's life.

If a patient cannot provide an answer or appears in distress, begin a detailed primary survey to identify life-threatening problems. You should be able to obtain a general impression of the patient's overall condition in a few seconds. This is also where your "gut feeling" comes into play and is something that, with training and experience, you should learn to rely on.

Exsanguinating Hemorrhage

In the primary survey of a trauma patient, you must immediately identify and manage life-threatening compressible external hemorrhage. If you are dealing with an exsanguinating external hemorrhage, it needs to be controlled even before assessing the airway or performing other interventions such as spinal motion restriction. This type of bleeding typically involves arterial bleeding from an extremity, but it may also occur from the scalp, at the junction of an extremity with the trunk (junctional bleeding), and other sites.

Airway Management and Cervical Spine Stabilization

Check the patient's airway quickly to ensure that it is patent (open and clear) and that there is no danger of obstruction. If the airway is compromised, it will need to be opened, initially using manual methods (trauma chin lift or trauma jaw thrust) (**Figure 2-3**), and cleared of blood, body substances, and foreign bodies, if necessary.

Eventually, as equipment and time become available and patient injury demands, airway management

Primary Survey Assessment

The primary survey of the trauma patient includes:

- General impression:
  - Clues to kinematics involved and potential for significant injury.
  - Patient positioning and any gross deformities.
  - Is there evidence of severe external hemorrhage?
  - Does patient appear awake and responsive?
  - Ask the patient's name and assess ability to interact.
- XABCDE:
  - *X (eXsanguinating hemorrhage)*—Identify severe external bleeding through a rapid body scan.
  - *A (Airway management and cervical spine stabilization)*—Identify airway compromise or potential for this to develop; provide spinal motion restriction if indicated.
  - *B (Breathing)*—Identify breathing inadequacy or potential for this to develop. Observe and auscultate patient ventilation depth and rate; assess oxygenation with oximetry and maintain SpO_2 at or above 94%.
  - *C (Circulation)*—Palpate pulse points to estimate blood pressure (BP); assess skin color, temperature, and moisture to assess perfusion status.
  - *D (Disability)*—Identify neurologic dysfunction, assess level of consciousness using Glasgow Coma Scale (GCS), and observe pupil equality and assess their reaction to light.
  - *E (Expose/Environment)*—Identify significant injuries. Observe the entire body for signs of injury while maintaining normal body temperature.

This sequence protects the ability of the body to oxygenate and the ability of the red blood cells (RBCs) to deliver oxygen to the tissues.

Critical or Not Critical?

By rapidly assessing vital functions, the primary survey serves to establish whether the patient is presently or imminently critical.

CASE STUDY: PRIMARY SURVEY

- **X**—No exsanguinating hemorrhage.
- **A**—Partially obstructed, stridor.
- **B**—Breathing is slow and variable depth; lung sounds are clear and equal bilaterally; oximetry 95% on room air.
- **C**—Radial pulses are palpable; skin is normal color, warm, and dry.
- **D**—GCS 3 (E1, V1, M1) pupils are unequal (L:2, R:4); right pupil is unresponsive.
- **E**—Abrasions at right arm and right hip.

Questions:

- Has a life threat been identified?
- If yes, how does that affect the assessment process?
- How should you proceed with treatment?

When to Press and When to Pack

Direct pressure and hemostatic packing and dressings should be applied in cases of nonarterial severe bleeding in extremities and all severe bleeding from truncal sites.

can advance to include suction and mechanical means (oral airway, nasal airway, supraglottic airways, and endotracheal intubation or transtracheal methods). However, a simple and quick method should always be used first to make sure the airway is open.

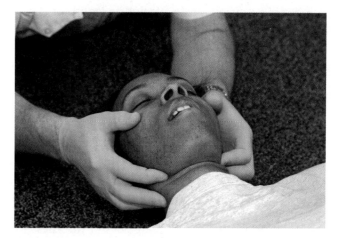

Figure 2-3 If the airway appears compromised, it must be opened while continuing to protect the spine.

> **QUICK TIP**
>
> Numerous factors play a role in determining the method of airway management, including available equipment, the skill level of the prehospital care practitioner, and the distance from the trauma center.

Spinal Stabilization

You should suspect that every trauma patient with a significant blunt MOI has a spinal injury until it is conclusively ruled out. When establishing an open airway, consider the possibility of cervical spine injury. Excessive movement in any direction could either cause or aggravate neurologic damage. The solution is to ensure that the patient's head and neck are manually maintained (stabilized) in the neutral position during the entire assessment process, especially when opening the airway and administering necessary ventilation.

This does not mean that necessary airway maintenance procedures cannot be applied. Instead, it means that the procedures need to be performed while protecting the patient's spine from unnecessary movement. If you need to remove a spinal immobilization device that was placed beforehand in order to reassess the patient or perform an intervention, you need to apply manual stabilization of the head and neck until the patient can again be maintained with spinal motion restriction.

> **QUICK TIP**
>
> It is particularly important to maintain a high index of suspicion for spinal injury in elderly or chronically debilitated patients, even with MOIs that appear to be minor.

Breathing

Once the patient's airway is open, the quality and quantity of the patient's breathing (ventilation) can be evaluated:

1. Check to see if the patient is breathing by looking for chest motion and feeling for air movement from the mouth or nose. If uncertain, auscultate both sides of the chest to evaluate lung sounds.
2. If the patient is not breathing, immediately begin assisting ventilations (while maintaining cervical spine stabilization in a neutral position, when indicated) with a bag-mask device with supplemental oxygen before continuing the assessment.
3. Continue assisted ventilation, and prepare to insert an oral, nasal (if no severe facial trauma), or supraglottic airway (if no signs of severe oropharyngeal trauma); intubate; or provide other means of mechanical airway protection. Also, be prepared to suction blood, vomitus, or other fluids from the airway.
4. If the patient is breathing, estimate the adequacy of the ventilatory rate and depth to determine whether the patient is moving enough air (minute ventilation = rate × depth).
5. Ensure that the patient is not hypoxic and that the oxygen saturation is greater than or equal to 94%. Provide supplemental oxygen (and assisted ventilation) as needed to maintain an adequate oxygen saturation.
6. If the patient is conscious, listen to the patient talk to assess whether they can speak a full sentence without difficulty. Also note any airway sounds that you may hear as they speak (i.e., raspy voice, stridor, wheezing).

> **QUICK TIP**
>
> Do not allow an advanced airway procedure to increase your scene time. If the procedure can be accomplished in the back of the ambulance, perform it there.

> **It Takes Your Breath Away**
>
> Injuries that may impede ventilation include:
>
> - Tension pneumothorax
> - Flail chest
> - Spinal cord injuries
> - Traumatic brain injuries
>
> These injuries should be identified or suspected during the primary survey and require that ventilatory support be initiated at once.
> Needle decompression should be performed immediately if tension pneumothorax is suspected.

Circulation

Assessing for circulatory system compromise or failure is the next step in caring for the trauma patient. Oxygenation of the RBCs without delivery to the tissue cells is of no benefit to the patient. After assessing the patient's airway and breathing status, you can get an adequate overall estimate of the patient's cardiac output and perfusion status. Hemorrhage—either external or internal—is the most common cause of preventable death from trauma. The patient's overall circulatory status can be determined by checking peripheral pulses and evaluating skin color, temperature, and moisture.

> **QUICK TIP**
>
> Assessment of perfusion may be challenging in geriatric or pediatric patients or in those who are well conditioned or taking certain medications (such as beta blockers). Shock in trauma patients is almost always due to external or internal hemorrhage.

Evaluate the pulse for presence, quality, and regularity. A quick check of the pulse will reveal whether the patient has tachycardia, bradycardia, or an irregular rhythm.

In the primary survey, determination of an exact pulse rate is not necessary. Instead, quickly get a rough estimate, and obtain the actual pulse rate later in the process. In trauma patients, it is important to

> **QUICK TIP**
>
> Although the absence of peripheral pulses in the presence of central pulses usually represents profound hypotension, the presence of peripheral pulses should not be overly reassuring.

> **Caution**
>
> **Pulse Pressure Association**
>
> In the past, the presence of a radial pulse was thought to indicate a systolic blood pressure of at least 80 mm Hg, with the presence of a femoral pulse indicating blood pressure of at least 70 mm Hg, and presence of only a carotid pulse indicating blood pressure of 60 mm Hg. Evidence has shown this theory to be inaccurate; it actually overestimates blood pressures. It can, however, be considered a good assessment of peripheral perfusion.

consider treatable causes of abnormal vital signs and physical findings.

Disability

The next step in the primary survey is assessment of nervous system function (including the spinal cord). This begins with determining the patient's level of consciousness (LOC).

You should assume that a confused, belligerent, combative, or uncooperative patient is hypoxic or has suffered a traumatic brain injury (TBI) until proved otherwise. Most patients want help when their lives are medically threatened. If a patient refuses help, you need to consider why. Does the patient feel threatened? If so, further attempts to establish rapport can help gain the patient's trust. If nothing in the situation seems to be threatening, the source of the behavior may be physiologic, and reversible conditions need to be identified and treated.

During the assessment, the history can help determine whether the patient lost consciousness at any time since the injury occurred, whether toxic substances might be involved (and what they might be), and whether the patient has any preexisting conditions that may produce a decreased LOC or aberrant behavior. Careful observation of the scene can provide invaluable information in this regard.

A decreased LOC should alert you to the following possibilities:

- Decreased cerebral oxygenation (caused by hypoxia/hypoperfusion) or severe hypoventilation (CO_2 narcosis)
- Central nervous system (CNS) injury (e.g., TBI)
- Drug or alcohol overdose or toxin exposure
- Metabolic derangement (e.g., caused by diabetes, seizure, or cardiac arrest)

If a patient is not awake, oriented, or able to follow commands, quickly assess spontaneous extremity movement as well as the patient's pupils.

- Are the pupils equal, round, and reactive to light (PERRL)?
- Are the pupils equal to each other? Is each pupil round and of normal appearance?
- Does each pupil appropriately react to light by constricting, or is it unresponsive and dilated?

A GCS score of less than 14 in combination with an abnormal pupil examination can indicate the presence of a life-threatening TBI (**Figure 2-4**).

Quickly check the movements of the four extremities because they can provide very important materializing signs of injury. Do not miss a gross hemiplegia or paraplegia at this stage, because it has important consequences on spinal management.

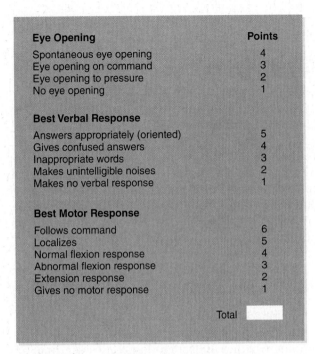

Eye Opening	Points
Spontaneous eye opening	4
Eye opening on command	3
Eye opening to pressure	2
No eye opening	1
Best Verbal Response	
Answers appropriately (oriented)	5
Gives confused answers	4
Inappropriate words	3
Makes unintelligible noises	2
Makes no verbal response	1
Best Motor Response	
Follows command	6
Localizes	5
Normal flexion response	4
Abnormal flexion response	3
Extension response	2
Gives no motor response	1
Total	

Figure 2-4 Glasgow Coma Scale (GCS).
© Jones & Bartlett Learning

> ## QUICK TIP
>
> Research has found that using only the motor component of the GCS—specifically, if this component is less than 6 (meaning the patient does not have voluntary motor control)—is just as predictive for severe injury as using the full GCS (see **Figure 2-4**).

Expose/Environment

An early step in the assessment process is to remove a patient's clothes, because exposure of the trauma patient is critical to finding all injuries (**Figure 2-5**).

Although it is important to expose a trauma patient's body to complete an effective assessment,

> ### You Can't Treat What You Don't See
>
> The saying, "The one part of the body that is not exposed will be the most severely injured part," may not always be true, but it is true often enough to warrant a total body examination. Also, blood can collect in and be absorbed by clothing and go unnoticed. After seeing the patient's entire body, you can then cover the patient again to conserve body heat.

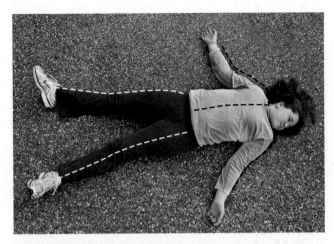

Figure 2-5 Clothing can be quickly removed by cutting, as indicated by the dotted lines.
© National Association of Emergency Medical Technicians (NAEMT)

hypothermia is a serious problem in the management of a trauma patient. Only what is necessary should be exposed to the outside environment. Once the patient has been moved inside the warm ambulance, you can do a complete assessment and then cover the patient again as quickly as possible.

> ## QUICK TIP
>
> Take special care when cutting and removing clothing from a victim of a crime so as not to inadvertently destroy evidence.

> ## FOR MORE INFORMATION
>
> Refer to the "Primary Survey" section of Chapter 6: Patient Assessment and Management in the PHTLS 10th edition main text.

Transport Considerations

If life-threatening conditions are identified during the primary survey, the patient should be rapidly packaged after initiating limited field intervention. Initiate transport of critically injured trauma patients to the closest appropriate facility as soon as possible.

Limited scene time and initiation of rapid transport to the closest appropriate facility—preferably a trauma center—are fundamental aspects of prehospital trauma resuscitation. Transport considerations include:

- *Destination decision*—The closest hospital that can provide definitive care may not be a trauma center but one that can manage a patient with uncontrolled bleeding or an unstable airway.

- *Duration and modality of transport*—Air transport may be available to provide faster and smoother transport to a trauma center.
- *Ongoing assessment*—Repeated assessment and continuous monitoring of the patient during transport.
- *Communication*—Notification to the receiving facility should be made as soon as possible. Early communication allows the facility to assemble the appropriate personnel and equipment necessary to best care for the patient, often by way of a trauma alerting system.
- *Prolonged transport*—In cases of prolonged transport, the crew must consider issues that concern the patient, the prehospital crew, and the equipment; for

example, the patient should be kept warm, equipment secured, patient vitals reassessed, treatments monitored, and the crew should use appropriate safety devices (e.g., seat belts).

National Guidelines for the Field Triage of Injured Patients

Correctly identifying trauma patients who are at high or moderate risk for serious injury is extremely important to avoid over- or under-triaging patients. The National Guidelines for the Field Triage of Injured Patients were established as a tool to help correctly identify the risk status of patients (**Figure 2-6**). Components considered are injury patterns, mental status and vital signs, mechanism of injury, and EMS judgment.

The guidelines use the following categories for patients:

RED—Transport to the highest level trauma center in the region.

YELLOW—Transport to a trauma center.

Use this approach to avoid over-triaging or under-triaging of patients. An example of over-triaging is transport of a stable trauma patient to a trauma center. Over-triage leads to reduced efficiency of patient care due to a large number of patients not needing specialty care. An example of under-triaging is transport of a critical trauma patient to a nontrauma center. Under-triage leads to reduced quality of patient care due to unavailability of specialty care.

Timing Is Everything

Keep scene time as brief as possible (ideally 10 minutes or less) when any of the following life-threatening conditions are present:

1. Inadequate or threatened airway
2. Impaired ventilation, as demonstrated by the following:
   - Abnormally fast or slow ventilatory rate
   - Hypoxia ($SpO_2 < 94\%$ even with supplemental oxygen)
   - Dyspnea
   - Open pneumothorax or flail chest
   - Suspected closed or tension pneumothorax
3. Significant external hemorrhage or suspected internal hemorrhage
4. Abnormal neurologic status
   - GCS score ≤ 13 or motor component < 6
   - Seizure activity
   - Sensory or motor deficit
5. Penetrating trauma to the head, neck, or torso or proximal to the elbow or knee in the extremities
6. Amputation or near-amputation proximal to the fingers or toes
7. Any significant trauma in the presence of the following:
   - History of serious medical conditions (e.g., coronary artery disease, chronic obstructive pulmonary disease, bleeding disorder)
   - Age > 55 years
   - Hypothermia
   - Burns
   - Pregnancy

CASE STUDY: TRANSPORT

A small community hospital is 10 minutes away, and the closest trauma center is 35 minutes away by ground transport. Air transport is available and, if requested immediately, can transport the patient to the trauma center in 14 minutes. The vital signs assessment is incomplete but there is enough information from the mechanism of injury and vital signs assessed to indicate the patient is seriously injured with a traumatic brain injury.

Questions:

- Where should this patient be transported?
- How should this patient be transported?

National Guideline for the Field Triage of Injured Patients

RED CRITERIA
High Risk for Serious Injury

Injury Patterns	Mental Status & Vital Signs
• Penetrating injuries to head, neck, torso, and proximal extremities • Skull deformity, suspected skull fracture • Suspected spinal injury with new motor or sensory loss • Chest wall instability, deformity, or suspected flail chest • Suspected pelvic fracture • Suspected fracture of two or more proximal long bones • Crushed, degloved, mangled, or pulseless extremity • Amputation proximal to wrist or ankle • Active bleeding requiring a tourniquet or wound packing with continuous pressure	**All Patients** • Unable to follow commands (motor GCS < 6) • RR < 10 or > 29 breaths/min • Respiratory distress or need for respiratory support • Room-air pulse oximetry < 90% **Age 0-9 years** • SBP < 70mm Hg + (2 x age in years) **Age 10-64 years** • SBP < 90 mmHg or • HR > SBP **Age ≥ 65 years** • SBP < 110 mmHg or • HR > SBP

Patients meeting any one of the above RED criteria should be transported to the highest-level trauma center available within the geographic constraints of the regional trauma system

YELLOW CRITERIA
Moderate Risk for Serious Injury

Mechanism of Injury	EMS Judgment

• High-Risk Auto Crash
  – Partial or complete ejection
  – Significant intrusion (including roof)
    • >12 inches occupant site OR
    • >18 inches any site OR
    • Need for extrication for entrapped patient
  – Death in passenger compartment
  – Child (age 0-9 years) unrestrained or in unsecured child safety seat
  – Vehicle telemetry data consistent with severe injury
• Rider separated from transport vehicle with significant impact (eg, motorcycle, ATV, horse, etc.)
• Pedestrian/bicycle rider thrown, run over, or with significant impact
• Fall from height > 10 feet (all ages)
	Consider risk factors, including:
	
	• Low-level falls in young children (age ≤ 5 years) or older adults (age ≥ 65 years) with significant head impact
	
	• Anticoagulant use
	
	• Suspicion of child abuse
	
	• Special, high-resource healthcare needs
	
	• Pregnancy > 20 weeks
	
	• Burns in conjunction with trauma
	
	• Children should be triaged preferentially to pediatric capable centers
	
	If concerned, take to a trauma center

Patients meeting any one of the YELLOW CRITERIA WHO DO NOT MEET RED CRITERIA should be preferentially transported to a trauma center, as available within the geographic constraints of the regional trauma system (need not be the highest-level trauma center)

Figure 2-6 Deciding where to transport a patient is critical, requiring consideration of the type and location of available facilities and the geographic restraints of the regional trauma system.

Secondary Survey

In the critical multisystem trauma patient, the priority for care is the rapid identification and management of life-threatening conditions. The majority of trauma patients have injuries that involve only one system (such as an isolated limb fracture). For these trauma patients, there is often time for a more thorough primary survey and a secondary survey. For the critically injured patient, you may not be able to conduct more than a primary survey. In these critical patients, the emphasis is on rapid evaluation, initiation of resuscitation, and transport to an appropriate medical facility. The emphasis on rapid transport does not eliminate the need for prehospital treatment. Rather, treatment should be done faster and more efficiently and possibly started en route to the receiving facility.

Because quick establishment of priorities and the general impression and recognition of life-threatening injuries are critical, you should memorize the components of the primary and secondary surveys and understand and perform the logical progression of priority-based assessment and treatment the same way every time, regardless of the severity of the injury.

The secondary survey requires a detailed head-to-toe examination to identify all injuries and conditions. As stated previously, it is only performed once the primary survey has been completed and all life threats have been treated. Vital signs are recorded and the SAMPLER assessment is performed.

See

- Be attentive for external or internal hemorrhage
- Examine all of the skin

- Note all soft tissue injuries
- Note anything that does not "look right"

Hear

- Note any unusual breathing sounds
- Note abnormal sounds auscultated

- Verify whether breath sounds are present and equal

Feel

- Palpate all body regions

- Note any abnormal findings

Figure 2-7 The physical assessment of a trauma patient involves careful observation, auscultation, and palpation (see, hear, and feel).

Eye photo: © REKINC1980/iStock/Getty Images; ear photo: © vvs1976/iStock/Getty Images; hands photo: © Image Point Fr/Shutterstock

© National Association of Emergency Medical Technicians (NAEMT)

QUICK TIP

Use your senses. When performing a secondary survey, use a "see, hear, feel" approach (**Figure 2-7**).

SAMPLER

- **S**ymptoms
- **A**llergies
- **M**edications
- **P**ast medical and surgical history
- **L**ast meal/last menstruation
- **E**vents leading up to the injury
- **R**isk factors for complications

Vital Signs

- Pulse rate and quality
- Ventilation rate and depth
- Oxygen saturation
- Temperature
- Blood pressure/mean arterial pressure (MAP)
- Consider blood glucometry if altered LOC
- Consider electrocardiogram (ECG) if trauma to chest or electrocution
- Monitor end-tidal carbon dioxide ($ETCO_2$) if advanced airway placed

Specific Patient Populations

Additional assessment considerations are required for specific patient populations.

- A geriatric patient (aged over 65 years [**Figure 2-8**]):
    - Language barrier
    - Hearing difficulty
    - Altered mental status
    - Comorbidities and medication effects
    - Less force in mechanism of injury required
    - Decreased airway protection

CASE STUDY: DETAILED ASSESSMENT

SAMPLER assessment is not possible. You assess the patient's vital signs. He is bradycardic, hypertensive, and has an elevated body temperature, which all suggest severe traumatic brain injury. Although altered LOC can be a sign of low blood glucose (BG), glucometry shows a BG of 100.8 g/dl (5.6 mmol/L), which rules out hypoglycemia.

Vital Signs:

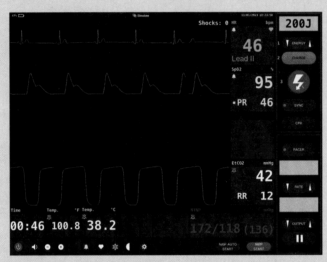

© National Association of Emergency Medical Technicians (NAEMT)

Secondary Assessment:

Detailed Physical Exam

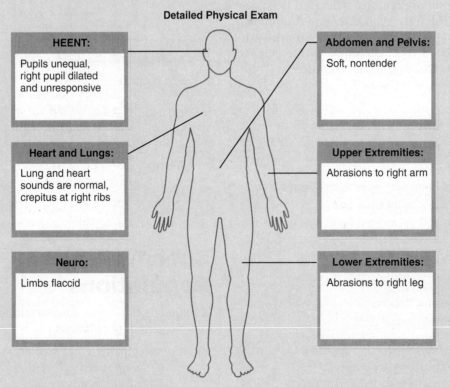

HEENT:
Pupils unequal, right pupil dilated and unresponsive

Heart and Lungs:
Lung and heart sounds are normal, crepitus at right ribs

Neuro:
Limbs flaccid

Abdomen and Pelvis:
Soft, nontender

Upper Extremities:
Abrasions to right arm

Lower Extremities:
Abrasions to right leg

© National Association of Emergency Medical Technicians (NAEMT)

Questions:

- Should the secondary survey be performed on scene or should transport be initiated?
- Will lack of SAMPLER information affect the patient care plan?

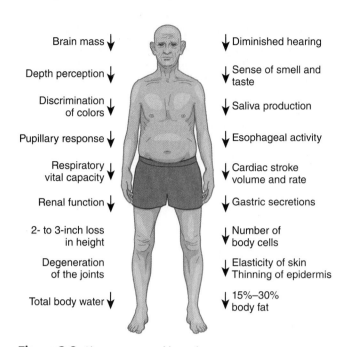

Brain mass ↓
Depth perception ↓
Discrimination of colors ↓
Pupillary response ↓
Respiratory vital capacity ↓
Renal function ↓
2- to 3-inch loss in height
Degeneration of the joints
Total body water ↓

↓ Diminished hearing
↓ Sense of smell and taste
↓ Saliva production
↓ Esophageal activity
↓ Cardiac stroke volume and rate
↓ Gastric secretions
↓ Number of body cells
↓ Elasticity of skin Thinning of epidermis
↓ 15%–30% body fat

Figure 2-8 Changes caused by aging.
© National Association of Emergency Medical Technicians (NAEMT)

- Higher blood pressure may be needed for perfusion due to atherosclerosis
- Hydration status prior to injury
- Increased risk of abuse as causal factor
- Positioning and stabilization or immobilization may need to be modified due to anatomical abnormalities
- Inability to maintain body temperature
- A pediatric patient (aged under 8 years):
  - Increased oxygen demand
  - Increased loss of body heat
  - Abdominal organs are poorly protected against blunt trauma
  - Lung injury can occur without associated rib injury
  - More susceptible to airway occlusion
  - Difficulty understanding, fear
  - Mechanism of injury unlike that for adult patient
  - Specialized equipment needed—stethoscope, BP cuff, oximetry probe
  - Modify the GCS scale
  - Increased risk of abuse as causal factor
- A pregnant patient:
  - Physiological changes: decreased cardiac output, relative anemia, supine hypotension syndrome, increased oxygen demand, decreased functional residual lung capacity
  - Increased pressure on internal organs
  - Increased risk of trauma
  - Less force to thorax required to cause injury

- A bariatric patient:
  - Increased tissue may impact ability for auscultation, palpation, and inspection.
  - Transport logistics will be more complicated and can interfere with assessment.
  - Specialized equipment may be needed.
  - At greater risk for heat illness.

CASE STUDY: WRAP-UP

The patient was transported to a Level I trauma center, where CT showed a subarachnoid hemorrhage with right temporal and right parietal subdural hematoma and cerebral edema; x-ray studies showed three fractured right ribs. The patient was admitted, hypertonic IV solution was administered, and a right-sided decompressive craniectomy was performed to address the edema and increased intracranial pressure (ICP). He was discharged home after six months of rehab.

Traumatic Cardiac Arrest Principles of Care

Do not treat traumatic cardiac arrest in the same manner as medical cardiac arrest. Priority should be placed on reversible causes—for example, stopping severe bleeding before restoring circulation with CPR. Take the time to correct reversible causes of cardiac arrest prior to transport, such as performing chest decompression.

If cardiac arrest occurs within 15 minutes or less of EMS arrival or is witnessed by EMS, consider immediate transport and begin resuscitation attempts en route to definitive care. Always follow local protocols.

If the mechanism of injury does not seem significant enough to have caused cardiac arrest, consider whether the patient may have suffered a medical cardiac arrest prior to the traumatic event (e.g., patient is in cardiac arrest after a minor MVC and otherwise appears uninjured).

Withholding Resuscitation to Patients in Traumatic Cardiac Arrest

Attempting to resuscitate a patient who is extremely unlikely to be successful exposes responders to

---

Traumatic Cardiac Arrest: Quick Check

- Resuscitation is attempted during assessment and while preparing for transport.
- Immediately control external hemorrhage.
- Prioritize reversible causes of cardiac arrest during resuscitation.
- Witnessed cardiac arrest (or occurring within minutes of EMS arrival) + transport time < 15 minutes = consider attempting resuscitation en route.
- Trauma may have resulted from a medical cardiac arrest.

---

unnecessary risk and commits high-value resources that could otherwise respond to a patient with a much better chance of recovery (**Table 2-1**).

Resuscitation may be withheld:

- In the presence of an obviously fatal injury such as decapitation or exposed brain matter

- If there is evidence of prolonged arrest such as rigor mortis, dependent lividity, or decomposition
- In the setting of blunt trauma and no signs of life, including apnea, pulselessness, and no organized ECG rhythm
- When there is penetrating trauma with no pulse, no breathing, no spontaneous movement, no pupillary response, and no organized ECG rhythm

Patient cohorts deserving special consideration before termination of resuscitation include:

- Pregnant patients
- Pediatric patients
- Drowning victims
- Hypothermic patients
- Patients in cardiac arrest due to lightning strike

Patients listed for special consideration include those who may, if there is no evidence of prolonged cardiac arrest, respond to a prolonged resuscitation attempt.

Table 2-1 Considerations for Choosing to Withhold Resuscitation in Traumatic Cardiac Arrest

Consideration	Presentation	Recommendation
Death is the most likely outcome even when resuscitation is initiated.	■ The patient is pulseless, apneic, lacks organized ECG activity, and has no spontaneous movement or pupillary reflexes.	Withhold resuscitation STOP
The injuries present are not compatible with life.	■ Decapitation ■ Traumatic separation of the torso (hemicorporectomy)	Withhold resuscitation STOP
There is evidence of prolonged cardiac arrest.	■ Rigor mortis ■ Dependent lividity ■ Evidence of decay	Withhold resuscitation STOP
There is evidence of a nontraumatic cause of arrest.*	■ Minor vehicle damage with a patient who appears uninjured ■ A fall from an otherwise nonfatal height without evidence of significant injury	Initiate resuscitation GO

*These are patients in whom there is suspicion that the traumatic event was a result of preceding cardiac arrest and not the cause of the cardiac arrest (e.g., falling from a ladder after suffering a major heart attack, crashing a vehicle after suffering a stroke, etc.).

© National Association Traof Emergency Medical Technicians (NAEMT)

Terminating Resuscitation to Patients in Traumatic Cardiac Arrest

Consider terminating resuscitation if the cardiac rhythm has deteriorated into a nonviable rhythm despite effective CPR, such as a narrow complex pulseless electrical activity (PEA) that has deteriorated into a bradycardic wide-complex PEA. If the duration of resuscitation exceeds 15 minutes, which is consistent with poor prognosis, you may also consider termination of resuscitation. Finally, consider termination of resuscitation efforts if the patient does not fit into one of the following categories: pregnant, pediatric, a victim of drowning, hypothermic, or in cardiac arrest due to lightning strike (**Table 2-2**).

The following are scenarios in which practitioners should *not* terminate resuscitation:

- Return of spontaneous circulation (ROSC) is achieved—discontinue CPR but continue resuscitation as needed.
- PEA is organized and consistent with producing effective circulation such as narrow-complex PEA that may be tachycardic or bradycardic wide-complex PEA.
- Patient may benefit from ED thoracotomy, such as a patient with penetrating chest trauma and with witnessed signs of life, or a patient with narrow-complex PEA with normal or tachycardic rate.

Table 2-2 Considerations for Terminating Resuscitation in Traumatic Cardiac Arrest

Consideration	Presentation	Recommendation
Signs of life are present.	■ Spontaneous respirations, movement, a pulse, or measurable blood pressure is present.	Do not terminate resuscitation. **GO**
PEA with organized ECG activity is present.	■ Narrow-complex PEA with normal or tachycardic rhythm (more likely to survive) ■ Wide-complex PEA with bradycardic rhythm (less likely to survive)	Do not terminate resuscitation. **GO**
The patient may benefit from ED thoracotomy.	■ Penetrating chest trauma with witnessed signs of life ■ Narrow-complex PEA with normal or tachycardic rate on ECG	Do not terminate resuscitation. **GO**
The patient is progressing into less-favorable ECG activity despite effective CPR.	■ Narrow-complex PEA with a normal rate decompensates into wide-complex PEA with a bradycardic rate.	Consider terminating resuscitation. **STOP**
The duration of resuscitation is consistent with poor prognosis.	■ Generally accepted to be no longer than 15 minutes. ■ Certain patient considerations may extend this 15-minute duration.	Consider terminating resuscitation. **STOP**

Abbreviations: CPR, cardiopulmonary resuscitation; ECG, electrocardiogram; ED, emergency department; PEA, pulseless electrical activity.

FOR MORE INFORMATION

Refer to the "Traumatic Cardiopulmonary Arrest" section of Chapter 6: Patient Assessment and Management in the PHTLS 10th edition main text.

Hemorrhage Control

External hemorrhage needs to be identified and controlled in the primary survey, because if it is not controlled as soon as possible, the potential for death increases dramatically. The three types of external bleeding are capillary, venous, and arterial (**Figure 2-9**).

- *Capillary bleeding* is caused by abrasions that have scraped open the tiny capillaries just below the skin's surface. Capillary bleeding is generally not life threatening and may have slowed or even stopped before the arrival of prehospital care practitioners.
- *Venous bleeding* is caused by laceration or other injury to a vein, which leads to steady flow of dark red blood from the wound. This type of bleeding is usually controllable with direct pressure. Venous bleeding is usually not life threatening but may be if bleeding is prolonged or a large vein is involved.
- *Arterial bleeding* is caused by an injury that has lacerated an artery. This is the most important and most difficult type of blood loss to control. It is generally characterized by spurting blood that is bright red in color. However, arterial bleeding may also present as blood that rapidly "pours out" of a wound or spurts out if a deep artery is injured. Even a small, deep arterial puncture wound can produce life-threatening blood loss.

Rapid control of bleeding is one of the most important goals in the care of a trauma patient. Nothing else can happen until external bleeding is controlled.

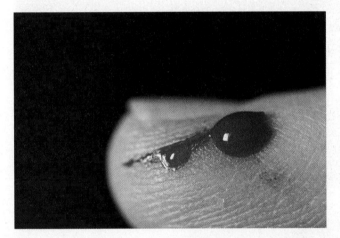

A

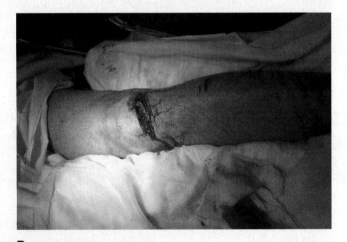

B

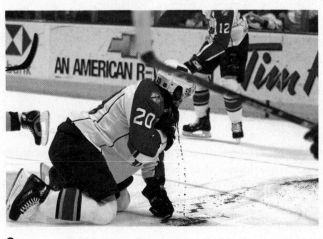

C

Figure 2-9 **A.** Capillary bleeding. **B.** Venous bleeding. **C.** Arterial bleeding.

Correcting Immediate Life-Threatening Bleeding

- Locate the source of bleeding.
  - Apply direct pressure to the source until bleeding stops.
- Use hemostatic dressings or tourniquets to stop bleeding.
- Avoid "popping the clot" and further diluting the blood through fluid resuscitation.
- Remember, all red blood cells count!

General Principles of Hemorrhagic Care

After the hemorrhage has been controlled:

- Keep the patient calm and at rest.
- Prevent movement of the injured region.
- *Do not* elevate the wound.
- *Do not* use pressure points.
- Preserve the patient's body temperature.
- Target maintenance of systolic blood pressure (SBP) to 80 to 90 mm Hg, or 90 to 100 mm Hg if traumatic brain injury is suspected.
- Provide supplemental oxygen to ensure adequate oxygenation of tissues despite loss of red blood cells.

QUICK TIP

The use of elevation and pressure on "pressure points" is no longer recommended because of insufficient data supporting their effectiveness.

General Principles of External Limb Hemorrhage Care

Hemorrhage can be controlled in the following ways:

1. *Direct pressure*—Direct pressure is exactly what the name implies—applying pressure to the site of bleeding. This is best accomplished by placing a dressing (hemostatic gauze is preferred) directly over the site of bleeding (if it can be identified) and applying pressure (**Figure 2-10**).
   - Apply pressure as precisely and focally as possible. A gloved finger on a visible compressible artery is often very effective.

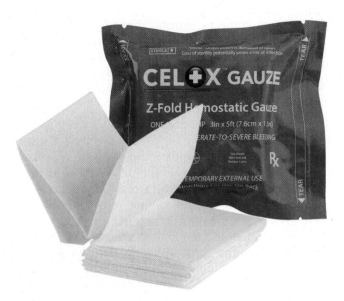

Figure 2-10 Hemostatic gauze is designed to be placed or packed in areas of the body that are not amenable to tourniquet placement.

QUICK TIP

If bleeding is not controlled, it will not matter how much oxygen or fluid the patient receives; perfusion will not improve in the face of ongoing hemorrhage.

- Combine direct pressure with wound packing and apply pressure continuously per the manufacturer's instructions for hemostatic gauze and for 10 minutes if using plain gauze. (This is the time required to form a clot.)
- Avoid the temptation to remove pressure to check if the wound is still bleeding before that time period elapses.

The application and maintenance of direct pressure requires all of your attention, preventing you from participating in other aspects of patient care. Alternatively, or if assistance is limited, a pressure dressing can be applied. Remember that application of pressure is a simple move that can be administered by a bystander, if necessary, provided there is an available pair of gloves.

2. *Tourniquet application*—Tourniquets are very effective in controlling severe hemorrhage when direct pressure or a pressure dressing cannot control bleeding from an extremity or if there are not enough personnel available

on scene to perform other bleeding control methods. In the case of life-threatening, or exsanguinating, extremity hemorrhage, you should apply a tourniquet instead of or concurrent with other bleeding control measures (**Figure 2-11**).

When placed correctly, a tourniquet compresses the tissue around the vessel to stop bleeding. Tourniquets must be applied tightly enough to compress tissue and muscles. No distal pulse should be felt if the tourniquet is applied correctly. If extremity bleeding is severe enough to be life threatening, tourniquets should be placed as proximal as possible (i.e., near the groin or axilla) on the affected limb as an initial measure to quickly gain control of the bleeding. If the bleeding site is readily and absolutely apparent, place the tourniquet 2–3 inches above the bleeding site but not over a joint

and tighten until the bleeding is controlled. You can also use other bleeding control measures, such as direct pressure and hemostatic agents, but they should not delay or take the place of tourniquet placement on an injured limb with severe arterial bleeding.

Occasionally, bleeding from distal or smaller arteries can be controlled with focused direct compression of the artery. However, this should only be performed if such bleeding can be controlled with a rapidly applied pressure dressing or if there is enough help on scene so that one practitioner can maintain manual direct pressure. If not, apply a tourniquet to the affected extremity.

A tourniquet cannot be applied to junctional wounds; thus, a device to control junctional bleeding is recommended if available (**Figure 2-12**). Packing with hemostatic gauze and placing a pressure dressing is an option if a junctional tourniquet is unavailable.

> **QUICK TIP**
>
> Regular training on tourniquet application is important. Use appropriate training devices and not devices intended for patient use.

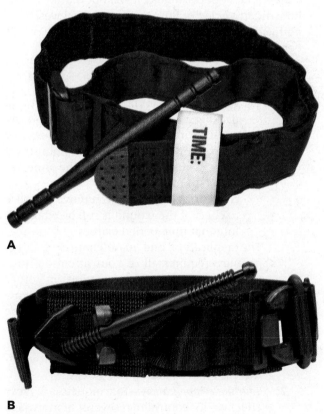

A

B

Figure 2-11 Types of tourniquets. **A.** C-A-T tourniquet. **B.** SOF-T tourniquet.

A: © Looka/Shutterstock; B: Courtesy of TacMed Solutions, LLC.

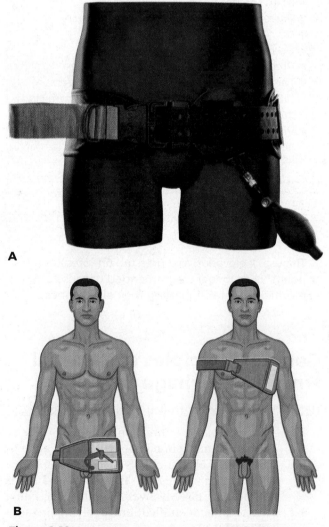

A

B

Figure 2-12 A. The SAM Junctional Tourniquet. **B.** Application of hemorrhage control devices at the junctional areas at the inguinal and axillae regions.

A: Used with permission from SAM Medical; B: © Jones & Bartlett Learning

In the Junction

Junctional hemorrhage is defined as bleeding that occurs at the junction of the torso with an extremity, including the base of the neck. Examples of junctional areas include:

- Buttocks
- Groin
- Axillae

The use of a tourniquet in these areas is often both impractical and ineffective.

General Principles of External Torso Hemorrhage Care

There are compressible and noncompressible sites on the torso. If the site is compressible, apply direct pressure to the source of bleeding. If the site is non-compressible, direct pressure can be accomplished by packing the wound with dressing (**Figure 2-13**). Intravenous administration of tranexamic acid can also assist with stabilization of wound clotting.

Internal Hemorrhage Assessment

There is the potential for massive internal hemorrhage in the pleural cavities, peritoneal cavity (which can hold a large volume of blood with little or no apparent

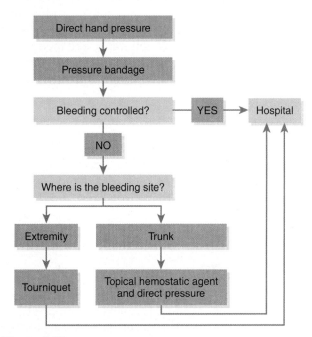

Figure 2-13 Hemorrhage control in the field.
© National Association of Emergency Medical Technicians (NAEMT)

abdominal distension), pelvis, and thighs—bleeding that cannot be controlled in the prehospital setting. Assessment guidelines include:

- Inspect the abdomen for bruising around the umbilicus or either flank indicating bleeding into the retroperitoneal space; however, these are rare and late findings.
- Inspect limbs for swelling and deformity.
- Palpate each abdominal quadrant to evaluate for tenderness, abdominal muscle guarding, and masses; tenderness and guarding can indicate peritoneal irritation due to the presence of blood.
- Gently palpate the pelvis for pain and instability, which suggest pelvic fracture with associated bleeding into the pelvic cavity.
- Palpate limbs for tenderness and deformity.

General Principles of Internal Hemorrhage Care

Internal bleeding requires hospital-based definitive care. EMS does not definitively treat severe internal bleeding—its role is to get the patient to definitive care. Internal bleeding management includes:

- Apply a pelvic binder if a pelvic "open book" injury is suspected. "Closing the book" will allow pressure to build up within the cavity and possibly tamponade the hemorrhage.
- Remember that external and internal bleeding can occur simultaneously. For example, in cases of traumatic amputation above the knee, the shearing forces that produce this type of injury commonly cause associated vascular damage and bleeding in the abdomen.
- If instability or pain is noted during any step of the examination, no further palpation of the pelvis should be performed and a pelvic binder should be applied.
- Splint any suspected fractures to prevent injury to blood vessels.
- Administer tranexamic acid IV to encourage clot stabilization at the wound site.

Transport Decision of Hemorrhaging Patient

Immediately apply direct pressure or a tourniquet to an exsanguinating hemorrhage. If you are unable to control hemorrhage, immediately begin rapid transport to a trauma center—the patient will exsanguinate before other life threats cause death. If hemorrhage is controlled, complete the primary survey prior to rapid transport to a trauma center.

During transport:

- Mitigate other life threats without delay and complete the primary survey if not yet completed.
- Support perfusion: keep the patient warm and at rest, initiate IV, and maintain minimal systolic BP (80 to 90 mm Hg, or 110 mm Hg if TBI is suspected).
- Provide supplemental oxygen.
- Administer tranexamic acid by IV.

Special Considerations of Hemorrhage Care

Patient populations with specific management considerations:

- Geriatric (≥ 65 years)
  - Decreased sympathetic response to low BP.
  - Decreased renal function puts patients at fluid overload risk with IV therapy.
  - Medication use may lower blood pressure, prevent sympathetic response to blood loss, and mask symptoms such as pain.
- Pediatric
  - Internal bleeding may be subtle.
  - Decreased volume loss required for hypoperfusion.
- Obstetric
  - Blood composition changes with gestation— blood has lower red blood cell count.
  - Increased oxygen demand due to fetus.
- Bariatric
  - Locating wounds and assessing for internal bleeding by palpation will be challenging.

Mass-Casualty Triage

A disaster is defined as a situation in which the number of patients presenting for medical assistance exceeds the capacity of healthcare practitioners with the usual resources at hand and requires additional, and sometimes external, assistance. This concept applies to all medical care settings, including hospitals and prehospital settings. This situation is commonly referred to as a mass-casualty incident (MCI).

QUICK TIP

The abbreviation MCI may also be used to refer to "multiple-casualty incidents," which are events involving more than one casualty, but may be handled with standard local resources.

When presented with such a situation, being able to effectively triage, treat, and transport patients in a timely manner can become overwhelming, so guidelines have been developed to aid in this process.

Triage is a process used to assign priority for treatment and transport. When emergency responders and medical resources are limited or insufficient for the number of injured, it is important to prioritize patients with the greatest chance of survival (**Figure 2-14**). The objective of mass-casualty triage is to do the greatest good for the greatest number of people with the resources available.

Corralling the Chaos

Mass-casualty triage in the field should be overseen by a trained triage officer. A triage officer should have a wide breadth of clinical experience in the assessment and management of field injuries, because potentially challenging decisions may be made about patients who are deemed critical versus those classified as mortally wounded or expectant.

START Triage

A number of different methodologies exist for evaluating and assigning the triage category. One method, the START triage algorithm (**S**imple **T**riage **A**nd **R**apid **T**reatment), involves a rapid physiologic and mental status evaluation (**Figure 2-15**). This system evaluates the respiratory status, perfusion status, and mental status of the patient in prioritizing casualties for immediate management (**Figure 2-16**).

QUICK TIP

Other triage systems include the MASS (**M**ove, **A**ssess, **S**ort, **S**end), SMART, JumpSTART (pediatric algorithm), and Sacco triage methods.

SALT Triage

The U.S. Centers for Disease Control and Prevention (CDC) convened a multidisciplinary group of experts and developed a consensus-based triage system, known as SALT (**S**ort, **A**ssess, **L**ifesaving interventions, and **T**reatment/transport).

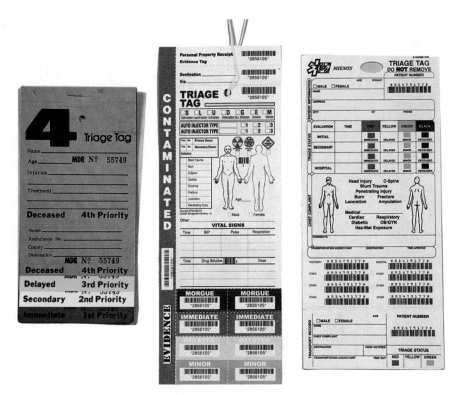

Figure 2-14 Examples of triage tags.
© File of Life Foundation, Inc

Triage Categories and Colors

Regardless of the exact triage method used, all triage systems ultimately classify patients into one of (usually) four injury-severity categories:

Highest priority patients are those who are identified as having critical, but likely survivable, injuries and are usually categorized as *immediate* and color-coded *red*.

Patients with non-life-threatening injuries (who may be nonambulatory) and can potentially tolerate a short delay in care are categorized as *delayed* patients and color-coded *yellow*.

Patients with relatively minor injuries, often referred to as the "walking wounded," are classified as *minimal* victims and color-coded *green*.

Patients who have expired on the scene or whose injuries are so severe that death is inevitable are categorized as *dead* or *expectant*, respectively, and color-coded *black*.

QUICK TIP

Some triage systems, particularly SALT, specifically separate those patients classified as mortally wounded from those who are dead, color-coding the expectant as *gray* (the rationale here being that expectant care does not mean no care).

This triage system involves sorting the patient based on the patient's ability to move, assessing the patient for the need for lifesaving interventions, performing those interventions, and ultimately providing treatment and transport (**Figure 2-17**).

It is important that triage personnel avoid the temptation to pause triage in favor of treating a critically injured patient. During this initial triage phase, medical interventions are limited to those actions that

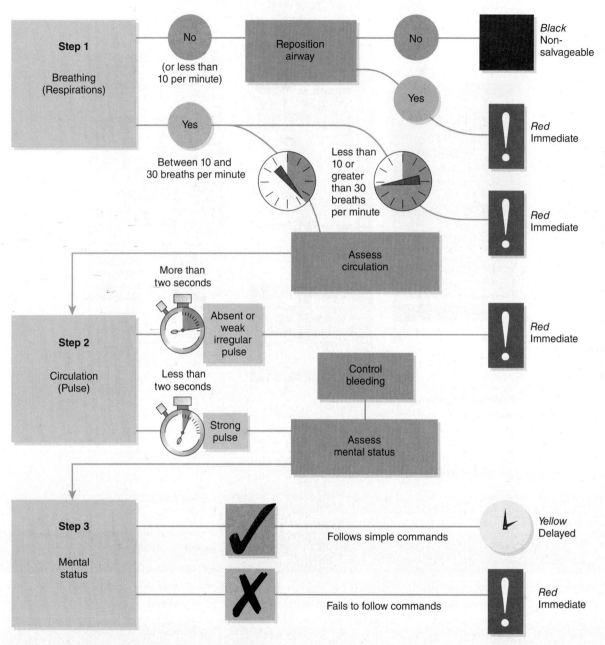

Figure 2-15 START triage algorithm: decision map.
Courtesy of Hoag Hospital Newport Beach and the Newport Beach Fire Department.

Respirations   **30**

Perfusion   **2**

Mental status   **CAN DO**

Figure 2-16 START triage algorithm: "30-2-can do."
Courtesy of Hoag Hospital Newport Beach and the Newport Beach Fire Department.

are performed easily and rapidly, and are not labor intensive. Generally, this means performing only procedures such as:

- Manual airway opening
- Administration of a chemical antidote
- External hemorrhage control, including wound packing and tourniquet deployment
- Needle chest decompression

SALT Mass Casualty Triage

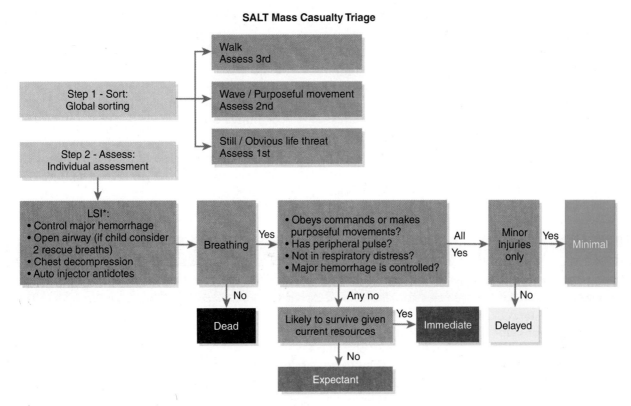

Figure 2-17 SALT triage algorithm. *LSI stands for lifesaving interventions.

Modified from Chemical Hazards Emergency Medical Management, U.S. Department of Health and Human Services. SALT mass casualty triage algorithm (sort, assess, lifesaving interventions, treatment/transport). Accessed December 14, 2021. https://chemm.hhs.gov/salttriage.htm

Interventions such as bag-mask ventilation, closed chest compression, establishing IV access, and endotracheal intubation are often deferred during the triage process. Generally, any intervention that immobilizes the practitioner should be avoided.

> **FOR MORE INFORMATION**
>
> *Refer to the "Patient Assessment and Triage" section of Chapter 5: Scene Management in the PHTLS 10th edition main text.*

SUMMARY

- Scene safety of prehospital care practitioners and the patient is the priority.

- Perform the primary survey to identify life threats.

- Hemorrhage must always be managed before all other life threats.

- All life threats are to be managed as soon as discovered after hemorrhage is under control.

- Utilize the National Field Triage Guidelines to make prehospital transport decisions to avoid over- or under-triaging patients.

- Transport considerations include the destination decision, duration and modality of transport, ongoing assessment, and considerations of prolonged transport. Use the secondary assessment and detailed assessment to identify all injuries and conditions only *after* all life threats have been treated.

- Do not treat traumatic cardiac arrest in the same manner as medical cardiac arrest. Priority should be placed on reversible causes.

- Attempting to resuscitate a patient who is extremely unlikely to be successful exposes responders to unnecessary risk and commits high value resources that could otherwise respond to a patient with much better chance of recovery.

- Hemorrhagic control in the field involves locating the source of bleeding, applying direct pressure to the source until bleeding stops, use of hemostatic dressings or tourniquets to stop bleeding, and avoiding "popping the clot" and further diluting the blood through fluid resuscitation.

- When properly applied, a tourniquet compresses the tissue around the vessel to stop bleeding.

Tourniquets must be applied high above the bleeding site and tightly enough to compress tissue and muscles. A standard tourniquet cannot be applied to junctional wounds.

- Massive internal hemorrhage cannot be treated in the prehospital setting. Transport immediately to definitive care.

- Triage, especially in the mass casualty setting, is one of the most important missions of any disaster medical response.

CASE STUDY RECAP

Dispatch

What scene safety concerns or considerations are present?	▪ Visibility ▪ Road surface traction ▪ Amount of traffic ▪ Risk of lightning or high winds ▪ Location of patient (on roadway?) ▪ Air temperature
What other patient-related information would you like to know?	▪ Was the patient wearing a helmet? ▪ What was the speed of the car? ▪ How was the cyclist struck (i.e., from behind or the side)? ▪ Did the patient hit anything else? ▪ What might be wrong with the patient? ▪ What is the transport time to a local trauma center? ▪ Is air transport available and appropriate?

Initial Impression

Remembering your priorities of care and the importance of scene safety, what are potential scene hazards?	▪ Body fluid and body fluid–contaminated clothing and debris ▪ Slippery surface ▪ Reduced visibility ▪ High speed traffic ▪ Road design such as lanes too narrow or scene hidden by a rise in the road ▪ Sharp-edged debris ▪ Trip hazards ▪ Poor lighting
What methods can you use to mitigate these scene hazards?	▪ Use of PPE ▪ Reflective clothing ▪ Vehicle positioning to block traffic and add light to scene ▪ Use of law enforcement officers to control traffic ▪ Use of traffic cones or warning signs ▪ Three points of contact when exiting a vehicle ▪ Coordinating scene activities such as moving the patient with other responders ▪ Removing trip hazards

| Are additional resources needed? | ■ Take into consideration whether there is any indication for launching a helicopter to assist with transport. |
| Can the patient be assessed in the prone position? | ■ No. While maintaining the spine in neutral position, the patient is placed supine for assessment. |

Primary Survey	
Is a life threat identified?	■ Partially obstructed airway. ■ The disability (D) assessment suggests a critical traumatic brain injury. ■ An unstable cervical spinal injury should also be suspected.
If yes, how does that affect the assessment process?	■ Note that the assessment continues after a life threat is corrected, such as the airway is maintained with jaw thrust and insertion of an airway adjunct.
How should you proceed with treatment?	■ This life threat cannot be corrected in the prehospital environment, so transport should be rapidly initiated.

Transport Decision	
Where should this patient be transported?	■ The patient is red according to the Field Triage Guidelines. A small community hospital is unlikely to have the specialized services required to provide definitive care to this patient.
How should this patient be transported?	■ Transport by air is reasonable due to the time saved to reach definitive care.

Detailed Assessment	
Should the secondary survey be performed on scene or should transport be initiated?	■ Transport should be initiated. A secondary survey should be conducted as soon as possible en route without delaying transport.
Will lack of SAMPLER information affect the patient care plan?	■ No

STUDY QUESTIONS

1. You are called to the scene of a possible mass casualty motor vehicle collision on the highway. Once you arrive on scene, what is your first priority?
   A. Immediately begin triaging patients.
   B. Treat the patient with the most visible blood loss.
   C. Determine the need for additional resources.
   D. Assess the scene and ensure it is safe.

2. A trauma patient from the highway incident is holding her right arm, and you note a significant amount of blood steadily flowing from a long gash. This is an example of what type of hemorrhage?
   A. Capillary bleeding
   B. Venous bleeding
   C. Arterial bleeding
   D. Road rash

3. What is the best way to control the bleeding?
   A. Direct pressure
   B. Elevation of the arm above the heart
   C. Tourniquet
   D. Occlusive dressing

4. The patient is wearing long sleeves, and you are having trouble visualizing the wound. What should you do?
   A. Cut the cloth away from the site until the entire wound site is visible.
   B. Leave the clothing in place. Put gauze over the wound.
   C. Remove the patient's shirt.
   D. Cut through the slash on the sleeve, and use the material as a makeshift tourniquet.

ANSWER KEY

Question 1: D
Ensure safety for responders, bystanders, and patient(s). The first consideration when approaching any scene is the safety of *all* emergency responders. When EMS personnel become victims, they not only can no longer assist others, but also add to the number of patients.

Question 2: B
Venous bleeding typically results in a steady flow of dark red blood.

Question 3: A
With venous bleeds, direct pressure is usually sufficient to stop the flow.

Question 4: A
Clothing can be quickly removed by cutting. You cannot treat what you cannot see.

REFERENCES AND FURTHER READING

National Association of Emergency Medical Technicians. *PHTLS: Prehospital Trauma Life Support*. 10th ed. Burlington, MA: Public Safety Group; 2023.

U.S. Department of Health and Human Services. SALT mass casualty triage algorithm (sort, assess, lifesaving interventions, treatment/transport). https://chemm.hhs.gov/salttriage.htm. Updated September 1, 2022. Accessed November 7, 2022.

U.S. Department of Health and Human Services. START adult triage algorithm. https://chemm.hhs.gov/startadult.htm. Updated September 1, 2022. Accessed November 7, 2022.

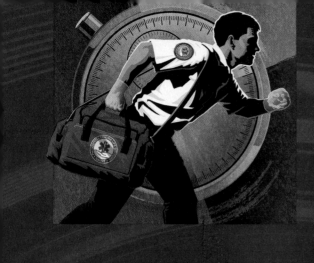

A—Airway

LESSON OBJECTIVES

- Discuss potential causes of airway obstruction in a trauma patient.
- Demonstrate assessment of a trauma patient's airway.
- Choose the most appropriate airway management intervention based on the patient's physical findings.
- Describe the structural differences in the airway anatomy of adult, pediatric, and geriatric patients.
- Discuss airway management considerations for pediatric and geriatric trauma patients.

Introduction

Two of the most important things you need to know in the prehospital setting are to provide and maintain airway patency and pulmonary ventilation. The failure to adequately ventilate a trauma patient and maintain oxygenation of organs causes additional damage, such as secondary brain injury. Ensuring airway patency and maintaining the patient's oxygenation and supporting ventilation are critical in improving the likelihood of a good outcome.

The respiratory system serves two primary functions:

1. Provides oxygen to the red blood cells
2. Removes carbon dioxide from the body

The inability of the respiratory system to provide oxygen to the cells results in anaerobic metabolism and can quickly lead to death. Failure to eliminate carbon dioxide can lead to coma and acidosis.

Anatomy

The respiratory system comprises the upper airway and the lower airway, including the lungs (**Figure 3A-1**). Each part of the respiratory system plays an important role in ensuring gas exchange—the process by which oxygen enters the bloodstream and carbon dioxide is removed.

Upper Airway

The upper airway consists of the nasal cavity and the oral cavity. Air entering the nasal cavity is warmed, humidified, and filtered (**Figure 3A-2**). Air entering the oral cavity bypasses these functions. The pharynx is next, and runs from the internal nares to the upper end of the esophagus. It is composed of muscle lined with mucous membranes and divided into three sections:

- The nasopharynx (upper portion)
- The oropharynx (middle portion)
- The hypopharynx (lower portion)

Below the pharynx is the esophagus, which leads to the stomach, and the trachea. At the junction of the hypopharynx and the trachea is the larynx (**Figure 3A-3**), which contains the vocal cords and the muscles that coordinate their function, housed in a strong cartilaginous box.

Directly above the larynx is the epiglottis, which acts as a flapper valve to prevent aspiration of solids and liquids into the trachea during swallowing.

Lower Airway

The lower airway consists of the trachea, its branches, and the lungs (see Figure 3A-1). On inspiration, air travels through the upper airway and into the lower airway before reaching the alveoli, where the actual gas exchange occurs. The trachea divides into the right and left main bronchi.

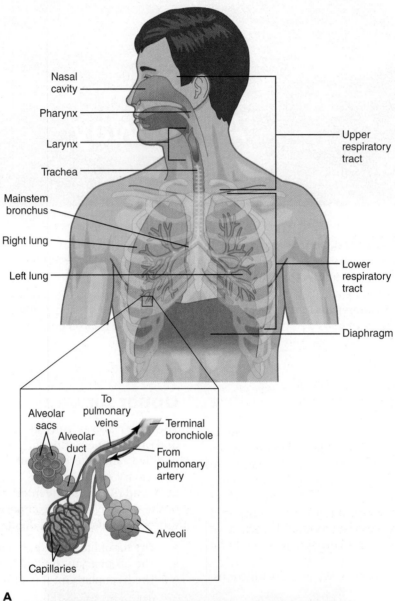

A

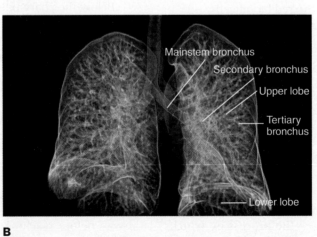

B

Figure 3A-1 A. Organs of the respiratory system: upper respiratory tract and lower respiratory tract. **B.** Cross-section of the lower respiratory tract.

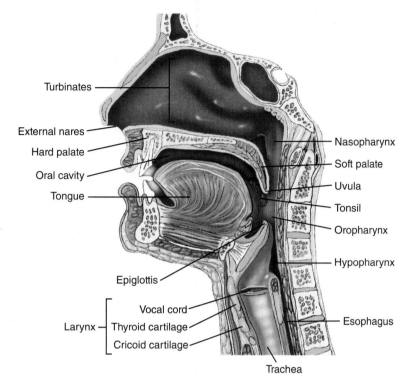

Figure 3A-2 Sagittal section through the nasal cavity and pharynx viewed from the medial side.

© National Association of Emergency Medical Technicians (NAEMT)

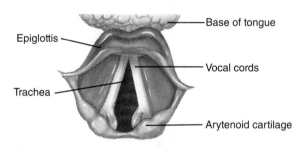

A

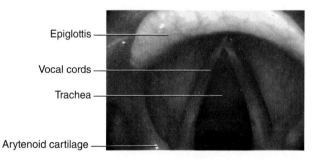

B

Figure 3A-3 Vocal cords viewed from above, showing their relationship to the paired cartilages of the larynx and the epiglottis. Unlike the upper airway, the larynx is made up of more delicate structures, including a thin mucosa and delicate cartilage, which are more susceptible to injury during therapeutic interventions.

A: © National Association of Emergency Medical Technicians (NAEMT); **B:** Courtesy of James P. Thomas, M.D., www.voicedoctor.net

Each of the main bronchi subdivides into several primary bronchi and then into bronchioles that terminate at the alveoli—the site of gas exchange where the respiratory and circulatory systems meet.

CASE STUDY: DISPATCH

You are dispatched to an older adult fall victim. The patient is an 86-year-old female. It is a cool spring day, 55°F (13°C), at approximately 1000. The patient was found by her daughter at the bottom of the basement stairs lying prone on the hard-tiled floor.

The fire department are first responders, and law enforcement officers are on scene.

A Level I trauma center is 30 minutes away by ground. The local hospital emergency department is 15 minutes away by ground.

Question:

■ What possible injuries to the patient do you expect given the scenario?

FOR MORE INFORMATION

Refer to the "Anatomy" section of Chapter 7: Airway and Ventilation in the PHTLS 10th edition main text.

Physiology

The airway leads atmospheric air through the nose, mouth, pharynx, trachea, and bronchi to the alveoli. When atmospheric air reaches the alveoli, oxygen moves across the alveolar–capillary membrane and into the vascular space, where it fills the O_2 bonding sites on the red blood cells (RBCs).

The circulatory system then delivers the oxygen-carrying RBCs to the left side of the heart to be pumped to cellular body tissues, where oxygen is used as fuel for metabolism. Carbon dioxide is exchanged in the opposite direction—from the bloodstream, across the alveolar–capillary membrane, and into the alveoli, where it is eliminated during exhalation (**Figure 3A-4**).

Assessment of ventilatory function always includes an evaluation of how well a patient is taking in, diffusing, and delivering oxygen to tissue cells. Without proper intake, delivery of oxygen to the tissue cells (and processing of oxygen within these cells to maintain aerobic metabolism and energy production) is impaired. If left uncorrected, anaerobic metabolism begins.

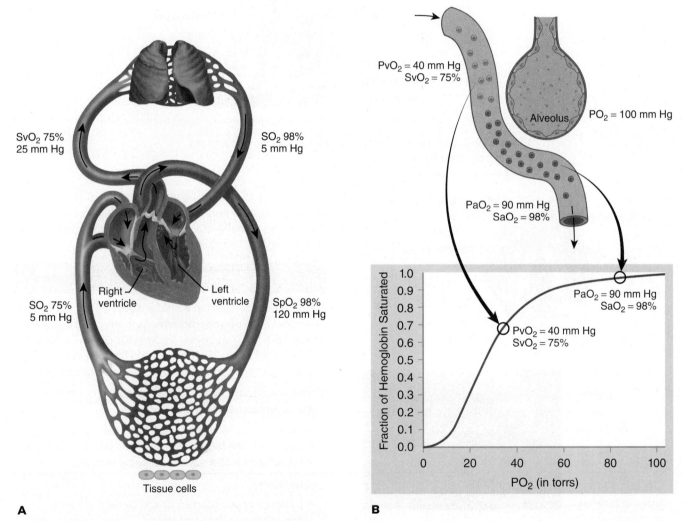

Figure 3A-4 **A.** Venous blood is drawn toward the heart via the low-pressure venous system (5 mm Hg in the vena cava just prior to entering the heart) and pumped by the right heart into the lungs (25 mm Hg after exiting the right ventricle). Oxygen is absorbed from the alveoli into the RBCs, while CO_2 dissolved in the plasma is excreted into the lungs. Fully oxygenated blood is then pumped in the high-pressure arterial system toward the body's tissues. **B.** As RBCs pass through the lung, they are exposed to oxygen molecules, which bind to hemoglobin molecules, resulting in the oxygen binding sites on the hemoglobin molecules becoming increasingly filled (oxygen saturation [SO_2] increases) and the partial pressure of oxygen within the blood (PO_2) progressively increasing.

Trauma can affect the respiratory system's ability to adequately move oxygen and eliminate carbon dioxide in the following ways:

- Obstructed airway, preventing movement of air into and out of the lungs
- Hypoventilation due to physical injury (e.g., rib fractures, pneumothorax, flail chest, head injury), resulting in diminished oxygen uptake and reduced carbon dioxide elimination
- Diminished oxygen uptake due to damage to lung tissue, as in lung contusion

Appropriate ventilatory support for all trauma patients begins by providing supplemental oxygen to help ensure that hypoxia is corrected or averted.

Just Breathe

Hypoventilation results from the failure of minute volume to meet increased demand. If left untreated, hypoventilation results in carbon dioxide buildup, severe hypoxemia, acidosis, and eventually death. Prehospital management involves improving the patient's ventilatory rate and depth by correcting existing airway problems and assisting ventilation as appropriate.

Hyperventilation can cause vasoconstriction, which can be especially detrimental in the management of a patient with a traumatic brain injury, and large tidal volumes can reduce venous return, which can be especially detrimental in shock patients.

FOR MORE INFORMATION

Refer to the "Physiology" section of Chapter 7: Airway and Ventilation in the PHTLS 10th edition main text.

Airway Assessment

You need to be able to assess the airway to effectively manage it. A patient who is alert and talking in a normal voice has an open and patent airway. But when the patient's level of consciousness (LOC) is decreased and exsanguinating hemorrhage has been addressed, it's essential to thoroughly assess the airway prior to moving to other lower priority injuries.

The primary survey is used to detect life threats. When examining the airway during the primary survey, you need to:

- **LOOK**
  - In the mouth for fluids or solids (vomitus, blood, broken teeth, dislodged dental appliances)
    - Use suction or manually remove the obstruction
  - For deformities or swelling of mandible and anterior neck
  - For abnormal chest wall movement; paradoxical movement, retractions, seesaw breathing
- **LISTEN**
  - For any abnormal sounds (stridor, wheezing, gurgling)

What's That Sound?

Upper airway sounds during inspiration are typically due to a partially obstructed airway. The type of sound you hear can give you some clues as to the cause and location of upper airway obstruction.

A gurgling respiration signals a patient's inability to clear and protect the airway and thus they are at risk of aspiration and/or airway obstruction with the next breath. This condition can be corrected, at least temporarily, by drainage or suction of the upper airway.

Although snoring, gurgling, and stridor sounds are all critical, stridor can be the hardest to manage. Stridor is a high-pitched whistling sound that can be heard on inspiration or expiration and can be caused by:

- Direct trauma
- Foreign body
- Swelling of the mucosa, as in inhalation burns

Airway Management

Airway management is a process. Assessing and properly managing a patient's airway to ensure the patient is able to ventilate is critical. Airway maintenance skills progress from basic techniques to advanced, with the application of these skills being patient-driven, dependent on the situation and the severity of the patient.

Manual methods of opening the airway are the easiest to use and require no equipment other than your hands. The airway can be maintained with these methods, even if the patient has a gag reflex. There are no contraindications for using manual airway management techniques in a trauma patient. Examples of this type of airway management include the trauma chin lift and the trauma jaw thrust. Positioning and manual clearing of the airway also fall into this category.

The first step in airway management is a quick visual inspection of the oropharyngeal cavity. Foreign material, such as food, pieces of a denture, or other small objects, and broken teeth are swept out of the mouth using a gloved finger; in the case of blood or vomitus, suction may be used.

In unresponsive patients, the tongue becomes flaccid, falling back and blocking the hypopharynx. Manual methods to clear this type of obstruction are easy because the tongue is attached to the mandible (jaw) and moves forward with it. Any maneuver that moves the mandible forward will pull the tongue away from the posterior hypopharynx.

QUICK TIP

Always weigh the risk versus the benefit of performing highly invasive complex procedures. These procedures require a high degree of skill proficiency and close oversight by the medical director. They should not be initiated unnecessarily, because the more difficult a skill is to perform, the greater the penalty to the patient for practitioner failure or error.

The Bariatric Airway

Bariatric patients need more oxygen for their increased metabolic demand, yet their lung capacity doesn't increase with their size. Keep in mind that a bariatric patient's normal respiratory rate may be much higher than the average adult's.

Airway Management Progression

Management of the airway can be challenging, but in most patients, manual or simple procedures may be sufficient—at least initially. Depending on the situation, these techniques can be applied immediately without any other material than your hands and lead to a better patient outcome than more complex techniques, which require increased time, personnel, and equipment, and have a higher risk of failure.

To manage the airway, you need to:

- *Assess*—Determine if the airway is open and if the patient can maintain a patent airway.
- *Position*—Many airway issues can be resolved by simple positioning or repositioning to open the airway and keep the tongue from obstructing the airway.
- *Suction*—Remove blood and secretions from the airway and clear any debris, broken teeth, etc., before inserting an adjunct or airway device.
  - *Adjunct*
    · Use the simplest adjunct in the most appropriate size needed to maintain the airway.
    · Use a nasopharyngeal or oropharyngeal airway before a supraglottic airway or endotracheal tube.
- *Ventilate*—Ventilate the patient if the patient is not breathing or not effectively ventilating on their own.
- *Oxygenate*—Administer supplemental oxygen as needed to maintain 94% or greater oxygen saturation rate (SpO_2) at sea level.

Positioning of the Airway and Patient

As you make visual contact with the patient, observe the patient's position. Patients in a supine position with a decreased LOC are at risk for airway obstruction from the tongue falling back into the airway.

An unresponsive trauma patient may be placed in the supine position on a vacuum mattress or backboard to achieve spinal motion restriction. Any patient exhibiting signs of decreased LOC will need constant re-examination for airway obstruction and the possible placement of an adjunctive device to ensure an open airway.

Position Matters

Patients with massive facial trauma and active bleeding may need to be maintained in the position in which they are found if they are maintaining their own airway. In some cases, this may mean allowing the patient to sit in an upright position. Placing these patients supine may cause obstruction to the airway and possible aspiration of blood.

The most common cause of upper airway obstruction is the tongue falling backward and obstructing the hypopharynx (**Figure 3A-5**). This causes airway

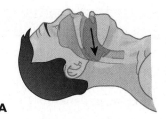 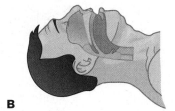 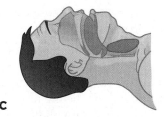

Figure 3A-5 Common causes of upper airway obstruction. **A.** Tongue blocking the airway. **B.** Vomitus, blood, or other secretions. **C.** Direct trauma to the larynx or inhalation injury.

© National Association of Emergency Medical Technicians (NAEMT)

obstruction along with snoring and abnormal thorax excursions, and in a trauma patient is often further complicated by blood and secretions in the upper airway. This can be corrected by positioning and simple airway maneuvers, such as the trauma jaw thrust or chin lift (**Figure 3A-6**).

- Use the trauma jaw thrust to open the airway and keep the tongue from blocking the airway. This allows for opening the airway with little or no movement of the head and cervical spine by a single practitioner (see **Figure 3A-6A**).
- The trauma chin lift uses two practitioners to open the airway. It maintains c-spine, and the chin is grasped to open the mouth and pull the chin forward (see **Figure 3A-6B**).

Once the airway has been opened, ventilations can be provided via bag-mask device (one- or two-practitioner techniques). Ventilate if patient's efforts to ventilate and oxygenate are absent or ineffective. Administer supplemental oxygen as needed to achieve oxygen saturation of 94% or greater.

Trauma Jaw Thrust

- In patients with suspected head, neck, or facial trauma, the cervical spine is maintained in a neutral in-line position. The trauma jaw thrust maneuver allows you to open the airway with little or no movement of the head and cervical spine.

Trauma Chin Lift

- The trauma chin lift maneuver requires two practitioners and is used to relieve a variety of anatomic airway obstructions in patients who are breathing spontaneously. The chin and lower incisors are grasped and then lifted to pull the mandible forward. Wear gloves to avoid body fluid contamination.

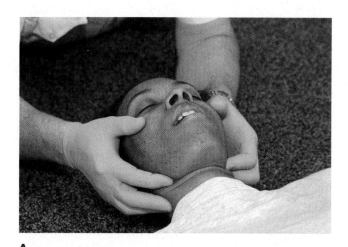

Figure 3A-6 A. Trauma jaw thrust. A thumb is placed on each zygoma, with the index and long fingers at the angle of the mandible. The mandible is lifted superiorly. **B.** Trauma chin lift. The chin lift performs a function similar to that of the trauma jaw thrust. It moves the mandible forward, displacing the tongue.

A: © National Association of Emergency Medical Technicians (NAEMT); **B:** © Jones & Bartlett Learning. Photographed by Darren Stahlman.

Positioning and Suction

Another common cause of airway obstruction is accumulation of secretions, blood, and debris in the hypopharynx when a patient is unable to maintain a clear airway due to decreased LOC or extensive trauma (see Figure 3A-5B).

- Logroll the patient and position on their side to facilitate clearing of airway.
- Use suctioning to remove blood and vomit from the hypopharynx before placement of an adjunct.
- If using a rigid large-bore suction device, introduce it laterally into the mouth. This approach is less stimulating and is better tolerated by a reactive patient. Prolonged suctioning can lead to hypoxia. Thus, once the airway is partially clear, hyperoxygenation may be performed.

Other Causes and Signs of Airway Obstruction

The third most common place of upper airway obstruction is the larynx, where obstruction can be caused either by direct trauma to the larynx cartilage or by inhalation burns with swelling of the mucosa (see **Figure 3A-5C**). This condition will manifest with hoarseness and stridor and usually will require an advanced airway, such as an endotracheal (ET) tube or surgical airway. You will need access to an advanced life support (ALS) unit or will need to expedite transport to the ED.

> ### QUICK TIP
>
> Swelling is a challenging situation because it occurs at the narrowest point of the upper airway. You must take steps immediately to alleviate the obstructions and maintain an open airway.

Limited chest rise can be another sign of airway obstruction. Additional signs, like the use of accessory muscles and the appearance of increased work of breathing during inspiration, should lead to a high index of suspicion of airway compromise.

When a patient is working hard to move air across an obstructed airway, negative pressure builds up in the chest, and you'll see retractions between the ribs and at the jugular notch when muscle and tissues are pulled into the chest. These retractions are especially visible in children. When the airway becomes even more obstructed, "seesaw breathing" or "rocking boat breathing" is likely to occur.

> ### FOR MORE INFORMATION
>
> Refer to the "Assessment of the Airway" section of Chapter 7: Airway and Ventilation in the PHTLS 10th edition main text.

CASE STUDY: INITIAL IMPRESSION

The patient's daughter had last seen her mother approximately one hour earlier, when she left to go to the supermarket for the patient. When she returned, she found the patient prone on the basement floor.

You assess the scene safety. There are 13 steps from the landing to the floor. There are two throw rugs, a half empty water gallon, and water scattered on the steps on the way down to the patient.

Law enforcement officers (LEOs) and fire department (FD) are on scene. FD first responders are in the basement with the patient. They moved her to a supine position and are holding manual c-spine.

You note a large pool of blood is on the floor next to the patient's head. There is a large hematoma on the right temporal area of the patient's head with active bleeding. Her right lower leg is obviously angulated and deformed. Patient is unresponsive with snoring and gurgling respirations.

Questions:
- What are the potential scene hazards?
- What life threats need to be addressed?
- Are any interventions needed before you proceed?

> ### FOR MORE INFORMATION
>
> Refer to the "Pathophysiology" and "Management" sections of Chapter 7: Airway and Ventilation in the PHTLS 10th edition main text.

Airway Adjuncts

Once the airway has been opened, airway adjuncts are used in conjunction with positioning to maintain airway patency (**Figure 3A-7**). The particular device should be selected based on your level of training and proficiency with that device and a risk–benefit analysis for the use of adjuncts and techniques relative to the patient. The choice of the airway adjunct should be patient driven, so ask yourself: "What's the best airway for this particular patient in this particular situation?"

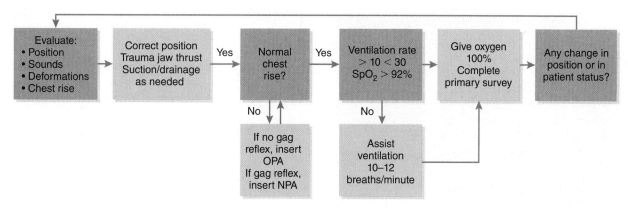

Figure 3A-7 Basic airway management algorithm.

© National Association of Emergency Medical Technicians (NAEMT)

There are several types of airway devices that may be selected depending on the needs or potential needs of the patient.

Simple Adjuncts

Simple airway management involves the use of adjunctive devices; the technique for inserting the device requires minimal training. The risks associated with these types of airway devices are extremely low compared to the potential benefit of maintaining a patent airway. Simple adjuncts are devices that lift the tongue from the back of the pharynx only. Examples of these airways include the oropharyngeal airway (OPA; **Figure 3A-8A**) and nasopharyngeal airway (NPA; **Figure 3A-8B**).

- Indications
  - Patient is unable to independently maintain their airway.
  - To prevent patient from biting an ET tube (OPA).
- Contraindications
  - OPA: Patient with an intact gag reflex
  - NPA: Possible basilar skull fracture (not an absolute contraindication, but caution is advised)
- Advantages
  - Quick and easy to insert
  - Can be used in conscious, alert patients (NPA)
- Limitations
  - Do not offer complete airway protection
  - Do not protect against aspiration
- Complications
  - NPA: Bleeding caused by insertion
  - OPA: Gagging, vomiting, and laryngospasm when used in patients with an intact gag reflex

Supraglottic Airways

Supraglottic airways, also known as advanced airways, are devices placed at the level of the oral pharynx and are meant to secure the airway above the vocal cords.

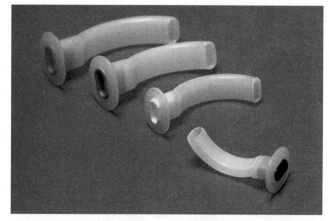

A

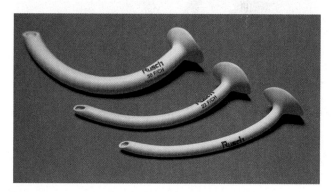

B

Figure 3A-8 A. Oropharyngeal airways. **B.** Nasopharyngeal airways.

© Jones & Bartlett Learning. Courtesy of MIEMSS.

They include the i-gel (**Figure 3A-9**), the laryngeal mask airway (LMA; **Figure 3A-10**), and the laryngeal tube airway (LTA; e.g., King LT).

- Indications
  - Airway maintenance in unconscious trauma patients who lack a gag reflex

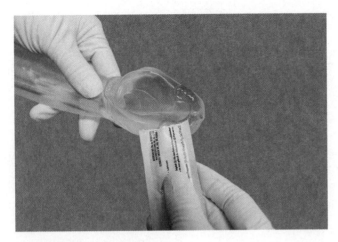

Figure 3A-9 I-gel ® device.

© Jones & Bartlett Learning. Photographed by Glen Ellman.

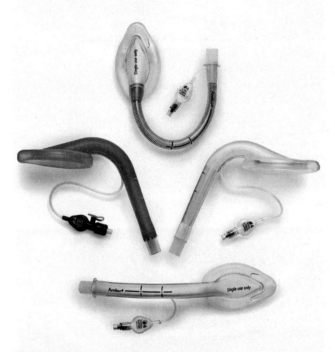

Figure 3A-10 Laryngeal mask airway.

Courtesy of Ambu, Inc.

- Useful in patients whose airway is difficult to maintain or who need positive pressure ventilation and with whom a tight mask seal is difficult
- Contraindications
  - Patient cannot have an intact gag reflex.
  - Can only be used in unconscious patients because it presses on the back of the throat.
  - Patients with known esophageal disease when using a King LT tube device.
  - Recent ingestion of a caustic substance.

- Advantages
  - Quick and easy placement (less than 20 seconds)
  - Excellent skill retention
  - May be inserted independent of patient position; for example, if there is difficult access to the patient or extrication difficulties
- Limitations
  - Does not offer complete airway protection.
  - Does not help laryngeal edema because it occurs distal to the terminal end of the SGA.
  - Esophageal seal can help prevent passive regurgitation, but the seal cannot withstand greater pressures, such as those generated during active vomiting.
- Complications
  - May cause gagging, vomiting, and subsequent aspiration.
  - Damage to the esophagus
  - If placed incorrectly, may cause hypoxia or hypoventilation.

Definitive Airways

Definitive airways provide the most effective protection against aspiration and airway closure by isolating the trachea from the esophagus. This is usually achieved by sealing or accessing the airway below the vocal cords. The risk of failure when performing a definitive airway technique is high. Examples of these airways include endotracheal tubes and surgical airways (cricothyrotomy). These are discussed in greater detail in Chapter 3B.

QUICK TIP

Continuous monitoring of oxygen saturation and end-tidal carbon dioxide ($ETCO_2$) is required when using supraglottic or definitive airways, adding to the complexity of their use.

Practice Makes Perfect

With complex skills such as intubation or surgical cricothyrotomy, the more times a skill is performed, the better the chance for a successful outcome. The more steps there are in a procedure, the more difficult the procedure is to learn and master. These complex skills also lend themselves to a greater probability of failure because greater knowledge is required and more steps are involved in completing the intervention. Generally, the more difficult a procedure is to perform, the greater the risk to the patient of failure or error. With airway procedures, this is particularly true.

It's All in the Timing

Transport time may be a factor; an example may be a patient whose airway is being maintained effectively with an OPA and bag-mask device with a short transport time to the trauma center. You may elect not to intubate but rather transport while maintaining the airway using simple airway techniques. Practitioners need to assess the risks versus the benefits when making the decision to perform complex airway procedures.

Airway Techniques Synopsis

Basic Techniques

Principle: In the normal state, the upper airway is open and the esophagus is occluded. Basic life support (BLS) airway maneuvers maintain the upper airway open so that air flows through the glottic opening into the lungs.

Specific Skills

- Positioning
- Suctioning
- Trauma chin lift, trauma jaw thrust
- Simple adjuncts: OPA and NPA

Can be used in a patient with a gag reflex (except OPA)

No airway protection against aspiration

Advanced Techniques

Principle: Isolates the airway so that air goes selectively through the glottic opening into the lungs.

Specific Skills

- *Supraglottic airway devices (i-gel, LMA, King Airway):* Occlude the esophagus while opening the airway.
  - Requires an unconscious patient
  - Offers only a little protection against aspiration
- *Endotracheal intubation:* Tube goes through the glottic opening into the trachea.
  - Requires a deeply anesthetized and relaxed patient
  - Protects the airway against both aspiration and occlusion through swelling
- *Surgical airway:* Tube goes through the cricothyroid membrane into the trachea.
  - Because it bypasses the pharynx and the glottis, it can be done in a conscious patient with local anesthesia or no anesthesia at all.
  - Protects the airway against aspiration.

FOR MORE INFORMATION

Refer to the "Selection of Adjunctive Device" section of Chapter 7: Airway and Ventilation in the PHTLS 10th edition main text.

CASE STUDY: PRIMARY SURVEY

Primary survey shows:

- **X**—Large laceration with active bleeding (blood pooling next to patient's head).
- **A**—Snoring respirations with gurgling heard in the airway; c-spine maintained manually by FD first responders.
- **B**—Slow, irregular pattern.
- **C**—Radial pulse is strong and regular.
- **D**—Unconscious and responsive to painful stimuli only. GCS 7 (E2, V2, M3).
- **E**—Supine on the floor; right lower leg angulated and deformed; multiple skin tears with bleeding noted on exposure.

Questions:

- Is the patient maintaining her airway?
- Is airway management indicated?
- What areas need to be addressed before moving on with the assessment?

Pediatric Airway Management

There are several anatomic differences that complicate the care of an injured child. Children have a large occiput and tongue and have an anteriorly positioned airway. Additionally, the smaller the child, the greater the size discrepancy between the cranium and the midface, and the large occiput forces passive flexion of the cervical spine (**Figure 3A-11**). These factors predispose children to a higher risk of anatomic airway obstruction than adults.

You should perform manual stabilization of the cervical spine during airway management and maintain it until a properly sized cervical collar is applied. Placing a 3/4- to 1-inch-thick (2- to 3-centimeter-thick) pad or blanket under an infant's torso can lessen the flexion of the neck and help keep the airway patent. Use bag-mask ventilation with high-flow (at least 15 liters/minute) 100% oxygen when the injured child requires assisted ventilation.

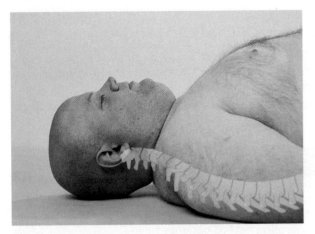

A

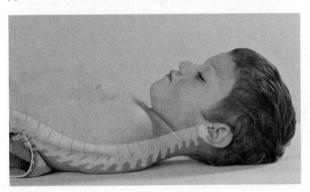
B

Figure 3A-11 A. Compared to an adult, a child has a larger occiput and less shoulder musculature. **B.** When placed on a flat surface, these factors result in flexion of the neck.

© Jones & Bartlett Learning. Photographed by Darren Stahlman.

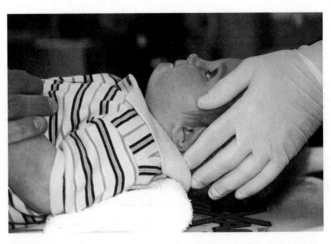

Figure 3A-12 Sniffing position.

© American Academy of Orthopaedic Surgeons

If the patient is unconscious, an oropharyngeal airway may be considered, but due to risk of vomiting, do not use it if the patient has an intact gag reflex.

Protect the Airway!

In the absence of trauma, a pediatric patient's airway is best protected by a slightly superior–anterior position of the midface, known as the sniffing position (**Figure 3A-12**).

QUICK TIP

Use a properly fitted oxygen mask and the "squeeze-release-release" timing technique. Watch for rise and fall of the chest, and if ETCO₂ monitoring is available, maintain levels between 35 and 40 mm Hg.

Consider the Epiglottis

When sized properly, the laryngeal mask and King LT airway are supraglottic airways that can be used for airway management in pediatric trauma patients who cannot be ventilated by a simple bag-mask device. In very young children, especially those weighing less than 44 pounds (20 kilograms), these devices can cause iatrogenic upper airway obstruction by causing the relatively larger pediatric epiglottis to fold into the airway.

In comparison to that of an adult, a child's larynx is smaller and is slightly more forward and toward the head (**Figure 3A-13**), making it more difficult to visualize the vocal cords during intubation attempts, so endotracheal intubation should be reserved for those situations in which airway management needs to be tightly controlled, there is impending airway obstruction, or there are insufficient resources to maintain effective bag-mask ventilation.

Psychological Trauma Needs Care, Too

Always consider the psychological considerations in treating a seriously injured child. There is an emotional impact while performing care. Although a proper debrief is necessary after a pediatric trauma call, do not force participation.

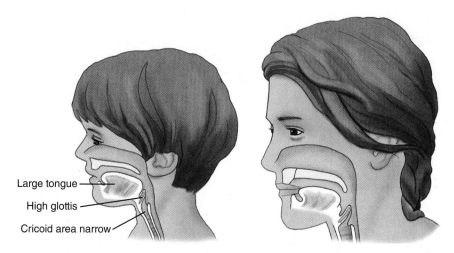

Large tongue

High glottis

Cricoid area narrow

Figure 3A-13 Comparison of an adult's and child's airway.
© National Association of Emergency Medical Technicians (NAEMT)

Caution

Nasotracheal intubation is not recommended in children because it requires a spontaneously breathing patient, involves blind passage around the relatively acute posterior nasopharyngeal angle, and can cause severe bleeding in children. Additionally, in a patient with a basilar skull fracture, it can inadvertently penetrate the cranial vault.

Surgical cricothyrotomy is usually not indicated in the care of a pediatric trauma patient, though it may be considered in a larger child (usually at the age of 12 years).

FOR MORE INFORMATION

Refer to the "Airway" section of Chapter 14: Pediatric Trauma in the PHTLS 10th edition main text.

CASE STUDY: DETAILED ASSESSMENT

SAMPLER assessment is not possible. You assess the patient's vital signs.

Vital Signs:

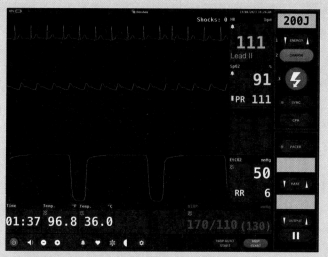

© National Association of Emergency Medical Technicians (NAEMT)

Secondary Assessment:

Detailed Physical Exam

HEENT:

(+) Airway gurgling.
Pupils unequal: left
dilated, right
constricted: large
hematoma to left
temporal with bleeding

Heart and Lungs:

Lung sounds – clear,
shallow, slow. Heart
sounds are normal,
no murmur.

Neuro:

Unresponsive
GCS 7 (E2, V2, M3)

Abdomen and Pelvis:

Soft, nontender.
Bowel sounds are
normal.

Upper Extremities:

Multiple skin tears
with minor bleeding

Lower Extremities:

Right lower leg
angulated and
deformed

© National Association of Emergency Medical Technicians (NAEMT)

Primary Survey Reassessment:

- **X**—Hemorrhage is controlled by a dressing and direct pressure.
- **A**—Held open with a trauma jaw thrust and NPA; C-collar in place.
- **B**—Patient is being ventilated with a bag-mask device at a rate of 10–12 bpm.

- **C**—Radial pulse is present and strong.
- **D**—Patient is unconscious and responsive to painful stimuli only.
- **E**—A scoop stretcher is used to remove patient from basement floor. Patient is placed on stretcher while maintaining spinal stabilization.

CASE STUDY: ONGOING MANAGEMENT

Questions:

- In this situation, when should the secondary survey, including vital signs, be performed?
- What are the management options for this patient?

- Is the patient stable or unstable?
- How will you manage the patient?
- How will you assess the adequacy of the patient's airway and breathing?
- Should a supraglottic airway be considered in this situation?

Geriatric Considerations

There are several physiologic considerations to keep in mind regarding the airway of a geriatric patient. Ventilatory function declines due to stiffening of the airway and decreased ability of the chest wall to expand and contract. The alveolar surface area of the lungs decreases

(4% for each decade after 30 years old). The presence of kyphosis, or change in the spinal curvature, produces ventilation difficulties, and stiffening of the rib cage can cause a reliance on the diaphragm to breathe (**Figure 3A-14**).

Other considerations include changes in mentation, which should not be assumed to be due to aging or dementia. Changes in mentation may be secondary to hypoxia from partial airway occlusion or obstruction. Also, remember patient position considerations (supine vs. 30 degrees).

Always examine the oral cavity for dentures or teeth that may have become dislodged or fractured.

- Dentures should be left in place to maintain a better seal around the mouth with a bag mask device.
- Dislodged or broken dentures should be removed as a potential airway blockage (**Figure 3A-15**).

Older adults may have an increased risk of hemorrhage from nasopharyngeal airway placement due to fragile nasal mucosal tissue and possible use of anticoagulants. Hemorrhage can complicate the airway and result in aspiration.

Early mechanical ventilation via bag-mask device or advanced airway measures should be considered because of greatly limited physiologic reserve.

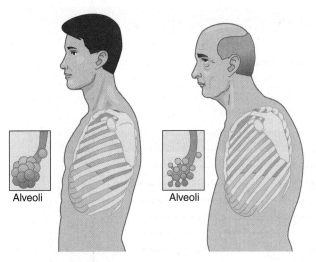

Figure 3A-14 Spinal curvature can lead to an anteroposterior hump, which can cause ventilatory difficulties. Reduction in the alveolar surface area can also reduce the amount of oxygen that is exchanged in the lungs.
© National Association of Emergency Medical Technicians (NAEMT)

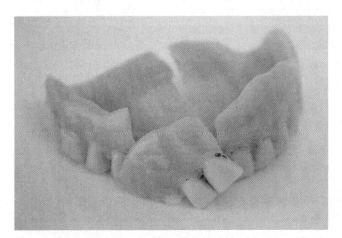

Figure 3A-15 Remove broken dentures to avoid a potential airway blockage.
© Leo Fernandes/Shutterstock

Geriatric Airway

Remember that a geriatric patient's ability to protect their airway may be compromised as the result of prior disease or cumulative exposure to environmental toxins caused by smoking or occupational hazards.

CASE STUDY: **TRANSPORT**

You decide to transport the patient to the nearest Level I trauma center, which is 30 minutes away, even though the local hospital is only 15 minutes away.

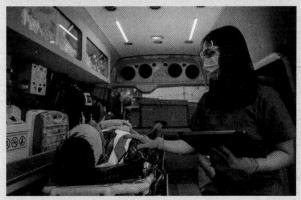

© ME Image/Shutterstock

Questions:

- How will you monitor the patient's airway during transport?
- Why are you transporting your patient to the Level I trauma center that is farther away than the local hospital?

CASE STUDY: **WRAP-UP**

The patient was transported to a Level I trauma center, where imaging showed a subdural hemorrhage. The patient underwent surgery to relieve the hemorrhage. The patient was discharged to a long-term care facility.

SUMMARY

- Trauma airway management can be difficult. Traumatic injuries can result in disruption of airways and structures.

- Start with the basics, then move to advanced management—if a simple adjunct or basic maneuver manages the airway, stay with it unless an advanced adjunct or technique is needed.

- Advanced airway techniques require repeated practice.

- Special populations like pediatric and geriatric patients require special airway management considerations, such as positioning.

- A failed airway renders all other trauma care fruitless. A patient with no airway will die regardless of any other interventions.

CASE STUDY RECAP

Dispatch

What possible injuries to the patient do you expect given the scenario?	Possible injuries include: ■ Airway obstruction due to trauma ■ Head trauma: Traumatic brain injury ■ External hemorrhaging ■ Other internal hemorrhaging

Initial Impression

What are the potential scene hazards?	Potential scene hazards: ■ Water on the steps ■ Throw rugs ■ Unstable or broken stairs
What life threats need to be addressed?	Life threats include: ■ Hemorrhage control ■ Airway compromise ■ Patient is unconscious and responsive to pain only
Are any interventions needed before you proceed?	Interventions: ■ Airway management ■ Bleeding control

Primary Survey

Is the patient maintaining her airway?	■ No. The airway is not patent. It needs to be repositioned.
Is airway management indicated?	■ Yes. Reposition and open the airway with a trauma jaw thrust, place a basic airway adjunct, and ventilate with a bag-valve mask to support ventilations.
What areas need to be addressed before moving on with the assessment?	■ Control bleeding from laceration. ■ Airway management including ventilations with a BVM and airway adjunct.

Detailed Assessment

When should the secondary survey, including vital signs, be performed?	■ Secondary survey may be delayed due to the presence of life threats and associated treatment. ■ If other EMS practitioners are present, secondary and vitals may be performed simultaneously with management of the life threats.

Ongoing Management	
What are the management options for this patient?	■ Continue the assessment. ■ Repeat and revisit the primary survey and interventions thus far. ■ Treat life threats.
Is the patient stable or unstable?	■ Patient has been stabilized with NPA, C-collar, bag-valve mask assisted ventilations, and control of bleeding
How will you manage the patient?	■ Continue to assess, reassess the life threat management, spinal stabilization, choose the appropriate destination, package for transport.
How will you assess the adequacy of the patient's airway and breathing?	■ Assess the adequacy of bag-mask ventilations, pulse oximetry, $ETCO_2$ reading, lung sounds, chest rise symmetry.
Should a supraglottic airway be considered in this situation?	■ A supraglottic airway is contraindicated in a patient with the ability to swallow. ■ Endotracheal intubation with pharmacologically assisted intubation/rapid sequence intubation (further discussed in Lesson 3B) could be considered for this patient. This is a time-consuming procedure, and the proximity to the trauma center, as well as whether bag-mask ventilations with basic airway adjunct are effective, should be considered.
Transport	
What type of facility are you transporting your patient to?	■ Level I trauma center due to significant head injury and airway compromise. ■ Neurosurgery capabilities are necessary.

STUDY QUESTIONS

1. You are called to the scene of an explosion and fire at a chemical plant where you find multiple casualties. Triage has begun. Your first patient is a 40-year-old man who was near the source of the explosion. He is unconscious and has extensive injuries. You note gurgling respirations. Why should you use the trauma jaw thrust maneuver first when dealing with a trauma patient?
   A. It's an easy technique that always works to open the airway.
   B. It allows you to open the airway with little or no movement of the head and cervical spine.
   C. Other techniques and interventions don't work as well.
   D. It can relieve a variety of anatomic airway obstructions in patients who are breathing spontaneously.

2. The patient becomes apneic. You suspect he has a cervical injury. Which type of airway should you use?
   A. Supraglottic airway
   B. Blind nasotracheal intubation
   C. Oropharyngeal airway
   D. Surgical airway

3. Why might it be more difficult to deal with an airway obstruction in a child?
   A. Children have longer tracheas.
   B. Children have larger heads and tongues so there is a greater potential for airway obstruction.
   C. Children have smaller heads, so there is less room to clear the obstruction.
   D. A child's epiglottis is smaller and stiffer than an adult's.

4. Why might you consider early mechanical ventilation via bag-mask device in a geriatric patient?
    A. Shorter tracheas in geriatric patients create the need for ventilation assistance.
    B. Laxity of the rib cage makes hyperventilation more likely.
    C. Geriatric patients have greatly limited physiologic reserve.
    D. Geriatric patients have a greater alveolar surface area of the lungs.

ANSWER KEY

Question 1: B
Manual maneuvers like the trauma jaw thrust or chin lift are always the first airway maneuver you should make when treating a trauma patient. In patients with suspected head, neck, or facial trauma, the cervical spine is maintained in a neutral in-line position. The trauma jaw thrust maneuver allows you to open the airway with little or no movement of the head and cervical spine.

Question 2: A
The supraglottic airway's greatest advantage is that it can be inserted independent of the patient's position, which may be especially important in trauma patients with high suspicion of cervical injury.

Question 3: B
Children have larger heads and tongues as compared to an adult so there is a greater potential for airway obstruction in a pediatric patient. You must pay special attention to the proper positioning of a pediatric patient to maintain a patent airway.

Question 4: C
Early mechanical ventilation via bag-mask device or advanced airway measures should be considered in geriatric trauma patients because of their greatly limited physiologic reserve.

REFERENCES AND FURTHER READING

Brown CVR, Inaba K, Shatz DV, et al. Western Trauma Association critical decisions in trauma: airway management in adult trauma patient. *Trauma Surg Acute Care Open*. 2020;5:e000539.

Carney N, Cheney T, Totten AM, et al. Prehospital airway management: a systematic review. Report No. 21-EHC023. Agency for Healthcare Research and Quality. https://www.ncbi.nlm.nih.gov/books/NBK571440/. Published 2021. Accessed April 22, 2022.

Kleine-Brueggeney M, Gottfried A, Nabecker S, Greif R, Book M, Theiler L. Pediatric supraglottic airway devices in clinical practice: a prospective observational study. *BMC Anesthesiol*. 2017;17(1):119. doi: 10.1186/s12871-017-0403A-6

National Association of Emergency Medical Technicians. *PHTLS: Prehospital Trauma Life Support*. 10th ed. Burlington, MA: Public Safety Group; 2023.

Warner KJ, Sharar SR, Copass MK, Bulger EM. Prehospital management of a difficult airway: a prospective cohort study. *J Emerg Med*. 2008;36(3):257-265.

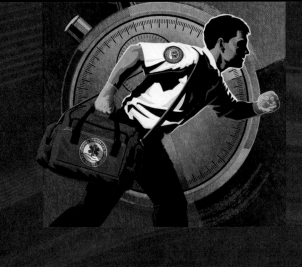

B—Breathing, Ventilation, and Oxygenation

LESSON OBJECTIVES

- Describe the physiology of breathing and ventilation.
- Discuss how trauma can impact ventilation and oxygenation.
- Recognize and treat tension pneumothorax.
- Describe management of a trauma patient's breathing, ventilation, and oxygenation
- Identify the equipment and assessments required to perform an endotracheal intubation.
- Describe how to maintain oxygenation and support ventilation in a trauma patient during prolonged transport.

Introduction

You already know how important it is to maintain the airway. The next step is ensuring adequate breathing (ventilation and respiration). Several factors can affect a patient's ability to breathe, especially when traumatic injuries are involved. These injuries can affect the respiratory system directly (collapsed lung) or indirectly (bruised rib causing pain and decreasing tidal volumes).

The thoracic organs are intimately involved in the maintenance of oxygenation, ventilation, perfusion, and oxygen delivery. Injury to the chest, especially if not promptly recognized and appropriately managed, can lead to significant morbidity.

Physiology

With each breath, air is drawn into the lungs. The movement of air into and out of the alveoli results from changes in intrathoracic pressure generated by the contraction and relaxation of specific muscle groups. The primary muscle of breathing is the diaphragm. Normally, the diaphragm muscle fibers shorten when they receive a stimulus from the brain.

In addition to the diaphragm, the external intercostal muscles help pull the ribs forward and upward. This flattening of the diaphragm, along with the action of the intercostal muscles, is an active movement that creates a negative pressure inside the thoracic cavity and causes atmospheric air to enter the intact pulmonary tree (**Figure 3B-1**).

> **QUICK TIP**
>
> Other muscles attached to the chest wall can also contribute to the creation of negative pressure; these include the sternocleidomastoid and scalene muscles. The use of these secondary muscles will be noticeable as the work of breathing increases in the trauma patient.

In contrast, exhalation is normally a passive process, caused by the relaxation of the diaphragm and chest wall muscles and the elastic recoil of these structures. However, exhalation can become active when air becomes trapped in the lower airways.

> **You Can't Get Negative Pressure in an Open System**
>
> Generating negative pressure during inspiration requires an intact chest wall. In the trauma patient, a wound that creates an open pathway between the outside atmosphere and the thoracic cavity can result in air being pulled in through the open wound rather than into the lungs. Damage to the bony structure of the chest wall can compromise the patient's ability to generate the needed negative pressure required for adequate ventilation.

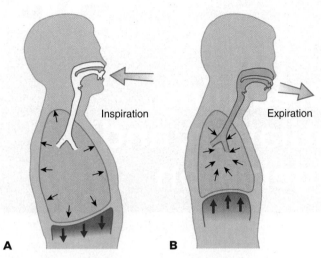

Figure 3B-1 When the chest cavity expands during inspiration, the intrathoracic pressure decreases and air goes into the lungs. When the diaphragm relaxes and the chest returns to its resting position, the intrathoracic pressure increases and air is expelled. When the diaphragm is relaxed and the glottis is open, the pressure inside and outside the lungs is equal. **A.** Inspiration. **B.** Expiration.
© National Association of Emergency Medical Technicians (NAEMT)

Assessing ventilatory function should include an evaluation of how well a patient is taking in, diffusing, and delivering oxygen to tissue cells. You need to ensure effective ventilation in your patient. Aggressive assessment and management of any inadequacies in oxygenation and ventilation are critical to a successful outcome.

Oxygenation

The oxygenation process involves the following three phases:

1. *External respiration* is the transfer of oxygen molecules from air to the blood.
2. *Oxygen delivery* is the result of oxygen transfer from the atmosphere to the red blood cells (RBCs) during ventilation and the transportation of these RBCs to the tissues via the cardiovascular system.
3. *Internal (cellular) respiration* is the movement, or diffusion, of oxygen from the RBCs into the tissue cells. Metabolism normally occurs through glycolysis and the Krebs cycle to produce energy.

Adequate oxygenation depends on all three of these phases.

When assessing a patient's ventilation, the first thing to look at is chest rise. You should determine if there's adequate and symmetrical chest rise and fall. You should look for three key parameters during the primary survey: ventilation rate, tidal volume, and

FOR MORE INFORMATION

Refer to the "Physiology" section of Chapter 10: Thoracic Trauma in the PHTLS 10th edition main text.

Components of Effective Breathing

For effective breathing, the following are necessary:

- A patent airway (to allow air flow)
- Ribcage and diaphragm in working order (to provide the mechanics of inhalation and expiration)
- A tight pleural space (to allow the lungs to inflate and deflate along with the movement of the chest cavity; fluid or air in the pleural space makes the mechanism less efficient)
- Two healthy lungs (to absorb oxygen)

symmetry of breath sounds. Look at the chest to determine if there is accessory muscle use and listen for any sounds. (Normal breathing should be quiet.) Bilateral auscultation should be used to check for a tight pleural space and determine the symmetry of ventilation and the presence and location of any abnormal lung sounds.

Technological advances, such as pulse oximetry (which measures the amount of oxygen in the blood) and capnography (which measures the amount of carbon dioxide being exhaled), can help with monitoring the effectiveness of our treatments; however, it's crucial that you always treat your patient and not the monitor—a patient showing a pulse oximetry of 98% but who is cyanotic needs treatment regardless of the oxygen saturation (SpO_2) reading!

Remember: A failed airway renders all other trauma care irrelevant, because a patient with no airway will die regardless of any other interventions.

Effects of Trauma on Ventilation and Oxygenation

Airway obstruction in the presence of altered mental status, broken ribs, air in the pleural space, paralysis of respiratory muscles, and/or unstable or perforated rib cage all cause a reduction of tidal volume. More complex oxygenation problems occur later in the ICU due to edema and inflammation but are rarely seen in the prehospital setting, so reduction of tidal volume (the size of each breath) is the primary concern in prehospital trauma.

In normal breathing, about 500 mL of air is taken into the lungs with each breath. As this air enters the upper respiratory tract, it first travels across the mouth, pharynx, and bronchi, which do not participate in gas exchange. The result is a volume of approximately 150 mL of that initial breath for which no air exchange takes

place, referred to as dead space. As such, only 350 mL of a "normal" breath is actually utilized by the body. Dead space volume also increases with large respirations.

The replenishment of the alveoli with oxygen-containing air, known as *ventilation*, is also essential for the elimination of carbon dioxide. Ventilation is measurable. The size of each breath (tidal volume) multiplied by the ventilatory rate for 1 minute equals the minute volume.

So, for the normal breath of 500 mL (tidal volume), at a ventilatory rate of 14 breaths per minute, the minute volume would be 7,000 mL/minute. However, we know that not all 500 mL reaches the lungs due to dead space, so we factor it in to the equation. Thus, tidal volume (500 mL), minus dead space (150 mL) provides us with a more accurate number for calculation. This gives us 350 mL × 14 breaths/minute equals 4,900 mL/minute or 4.9 L/minute, which is referred to as effective ventilation (**Figure 3B-2**).

Thoracic Trauma

Injuries to the thorax and its related structures are commonly seen in trauma patients; as with other body systems, these injuries can result from blunt, penetrating, or blast mechanisms. Thoracic trauma frequently

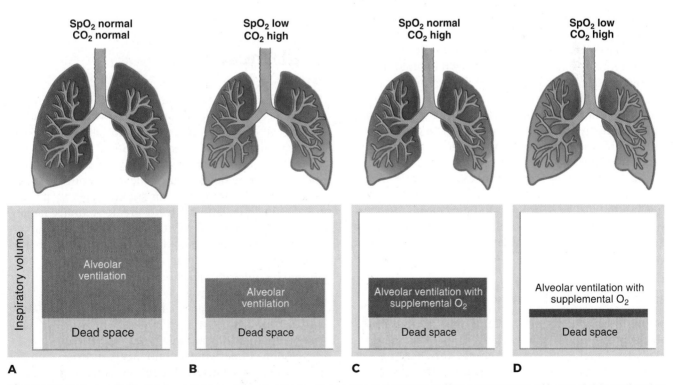

Figure 3B-2 As inspiratory volume progressively decreases, the ability to maintain sufficient saturation of hemoglobin molecules with oxygen decreases, and the ability to adequately clear CO_2 from the lungs is impaired.

impacts the respiratory system, via either direct injury to the lung itself or disruption of ventilation through injury to accessory muscles or the pleural space.

Penetrating Injury

With penetrating injuries, objects go through the chest wall, enter the thoracic cavity, and potentially injure the organs within the thorax. When a penetrating wound creates a communication between the chest cavity and the outside atmosphere, air can enter the pleural space through the wound during inspiration when the pressure inside the chest is lower than the pressure outside the chest. Air accumulates in the pleural space, decreasing the space available for the lung tissue and resulting in partial collapse of the lung. This prevents effective ventilation within the collapsed portion of the lung. Wounds that do not expose the pleural space can also be associated with lung collapse and accumulation of air in the pleural space when the mechanism of injury results in rupture of lung tissue or small airways. In these situations, pneumothorax results when air from the bronchial tree or from the lungs leaks into the pleural space with inspiration.

To make up for the lost ventilation capacity, the respiratory center stimulates more rapid breathing, increasing the work of breathing. The patient may be able to tolerate the increased workload for a time, but if not recognized and treated, the patient is at risk for ventilatory failure, which will be manifested by increasing respiratory distress as the carbon dioxide levels in the blood rise and the oxygen levels fall.

If there is continued entry of air into the chest cavity without any exit, pressure will begin to build within the pleural space, leading to tension pneumothorax.

This condition further interferes with the patient's ability to properly ventilate. It will also impact circulation negatively because venous return to the heart is reduced by the increasing intrathoracic pressure, and shock may ensue.

Lacerated tissues and torn blood vessels bleed. Penetrating wounds to the chest may result in bleeding into the pleural space (hemothorax) from the chest wall muscles, the intercostal vessels, and the lungs. Penetrating wounds to the major vessels in the chest result in catastrophic bleeding.

Blunt Force Injury

Blunt force applied to the chest wall is transmitted through the chest wall to the thoracic organs, especially the lungs. This wave of energy can tear lung tissue, which may result in bleeding into the alveoli. In this setting, the injury is called a pulmonary contusion. A pulmonary contusion is essentially a bruise of the lung. It can be made worse by fluid resuscitation. The impact on oxygenation and ventilation is the same as with penetrating injury.

If the force applied to the lung tissue also tears the visceral pleura, air may escape from the lung into the pleural space, creating a pneumothorax and the potential for a tension pneumothorax.

Blunt force trauma to the chest can also break ribs, which can then lacerate the lung, resulting in pneumothorax as well as hemothorax (both caused by bleeding from the broken ribs and from the torn lung and intercostal muscles). Blunt force injury typically associated with sudden deceleration incidents may cause shearing or rupture of the major blood vessels in the chest, particularly the aorta, leading to catastrophic hemorrhage. Finally, in some cases, blunt force can disrupt the chest wall, leading to instability of the chest wall and compromise of the changes in intrathoracic pressure, leading to impaired ventilation. Remember that ribs are more pliable in pediatric patients, and internal injury is therefore more likely.

> ## FOR MORE INFORMATION
>
> *For more information on thoracic trauma, refer to Chapter 10: Thoracic Trauma in the PHTLS 10th edition main text.*

Flail Chest

Flail chest occurs when two or more adjacent ribs are fractured in more than one place along their length. Consequently, a segment of the chest wall is in discontinuity, allowing the affected ribs to have paradoxical inward movement during inspiration when the ribs should move out and upward (**Figure 3B-3**). Initially, movement may not be noticeable due to muscle spasm and shallow breathing. In this situation, gently palpate for crepitus and auscultate to breath sound changes. The patient will present with pain, often severe; an elevated ventilatory rate; and avoidance of deep breaths due to pain. Hypoxia may also be present, as demonstrated by pulse oximetry or cyanosis.

Management of flail chest should focus on pain relief (narcotic analgesics may be used), ventilatory support, and monitoring for deterioration, especially the ventilatory rate and tidal volume. Patients who are developing underlying pulmonary contusion and respiratory compromise will demonstrate an increase in their ventilatory rate over time. Pulse oximetry is useful to detect hypoxia. Oxygen should be administered to ensure an oxygen saturation of at least 94%.

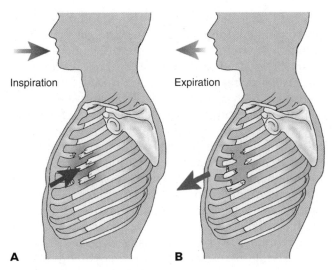

Inspiration   Expiration

A   **B**

Figure 3B-3 Paradoxical motion. **A.** If stability of the chest wall has been lost by ribs fractured in two or more places as intrathoracic pressure decreases during inspiration, the external air pressure forces the chest wall inward. **B.** When intrathoracic pressure increases during expiration, the chest wall is forced outward.

© National Association of Emergency Medical Technicians (NAEMT)

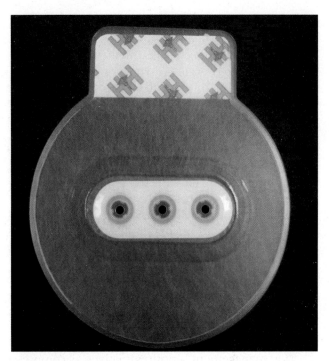

Figure 3B-4 Vented chest seals have been shown in animal studies to prevent the development of tension pneumothorax after sealing of an open chest wound.

Courtesy of H & H Medical Corporation.

Support of ventilation with bag-mask device assistance, continuous positive airway pressure (CPAP), or endotracheal intubation and positive-pressure ventilation may be necessary (particularly with prolonged transport times) for those patients who are having difficulty maintaining adequate oxygenation.

Open Pneumothorax

An open pneumothorax is caused by a defect in the chest wall that allows air to enter and exit the pleural space with each ventilatory effort. The process of air traveling into and out of the hole in the chest wall creates an audible noise; thus, an open pneumothorax may be referred to as a "sucking chest wound." Penetrating wounds result in an open pneumothorax only when the size of the chest wall defect is large enough that the surrounding tissues do not effectively close the wound during inspiration and/or expiration.

When the patient attempts to inhale, air crosses the open wound and enters the pleural space because of the negative pressure created in the thoracic cavity as the muscles of respiration contract. In larger wounds, there may be free flow of air into and out of the pleural space with the different phases of respiration.

Assessment of the patient with open pneumothorax usually reveals obvious respiratory distress. The patient will typically be anxious and tachypneic (breathing rapidly). Initial management of an open pneumothorax involves sealing the defect in the chest wall and administering supplemental oxygen. Seal

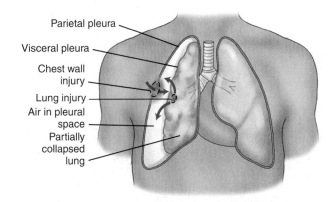

Parietal pleura
Visceral pleura
Chest wall injury
Lung injury
Air in pleural space
Partially collapsed lung

Figure 3B-5 Because of the proximity of the chest wall to the lung, it would be extremely difficult for the chest wall to be injured by penetrating trauma and the lung not to be injured. Occluding the hole in the chest wall does not prevent air leakage into the pleural space from the lung.

© National Association of Emergency Medical Technicians (NAEMT)

the chest wound with an occlusive dressing secured on three sides (or use a vented chest seal, if available [**Figure 3B-4**]) and administer supplemental oxygen. This prevents airflow into the chest cavity during inspiration while allowing air to escape through the loose side of the dressing (or vents) during exhalation, hopefully preventing development of a tension pneumothorax (**Figure 3B-5**).

Tension Pneumothorax

Tension pneumothorax is a life-threatening emergency. Tension physiology occurs when air or fluid accumulating in the chest cavity starts to compress the lungs, the great vessels, and the heart, blocking respiration and venous return (**Figure 3B-6**). If there is persistent entry of air into the chest cavity without any exit or release, pressure builds, ventilatory compromise increases, and venous return to the heart decreases. The decreasing cardiac output coupled with worsening gas exchange results in profound shock.

Initially, patients with tension pneumothorax will be apprehensive and uncomfortable. They will generally complain of chest pain and difficulty breathing. As the tension pneumothorax worsens, they will exhibit increasing agitation, tachypnea, and respiratory distress. In severe cases, cyanosis, apnea, and cardiac arrest may occur. Increasing respiratory distress with no breath sounds on one side is a sign of tension pneumothorax (**Figure 3B-7**).

The management priority involves decompressing the tension pneumothorax. You should perform decompression when the following three findings are present:

1. Worsening respiratory distress or difficulty ventilating with a bag-mask device
2. Unilateral decreased or absent breath sounds
3. Decompensated shock (systolic blood pressure less than 90 mm Hg with a narrowed pulse pressure)

Management of a tension pneumothorax in the prehospital environment is dependent on the clinical situation as well as scope of practice and local protocols. For instance, if only BLS-level practitioners are available, rapid assessment and safe, expeditious transport to an appropriate facility while administering high-concentration oxygen (fraction of inspired oxygen [FiO_2] $\geq$ 94%) is imperative. If the patient has an open pneumothorax with an occlusive dressing that has progressed to a tension pneumothorax, briefly opening or removing the dressing should allow the tension pneumothorax to decompress. If an ALS practitioner is available and the patient does not have an occlusive dressing, needle decompression (needle thoracostomy) can be lifesaving. Needle thoracostomy should be performed with a large-bore (10- to 16-gauge) IV catheter at least 3.5 inches (8 cm) long. The fifth intercostal space on the anterior axillary line on the affected side is the preferred site to potentially avoid injuring vessels and other organs. Be aware that this is a *temporary measure* and that pneumothorax can develop again. The patient should be rapidly transported to an appropriate facility. Intravenous access should be obtained during transport unless transport time is particularly short. The patient must be closely observed for deterioration. Repeat decompression en route may become necessary.

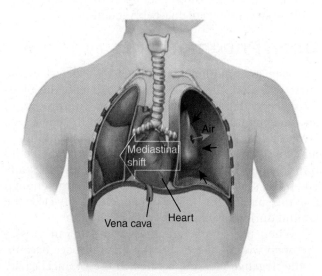

Figure 3B-7 Tension pneumothorax. If the amount of air trapped in the pleural space continues to increase, not only is the lung on the affected side collapsed, but the mediastinum is shifted to the opposite side. The lung on the opposite side is then compressed and intrathoracic pressure increases, which kinks the vena cava and decreases blood return to the heart.

© National Association of Emergency Medical Technicians (NAEMT)

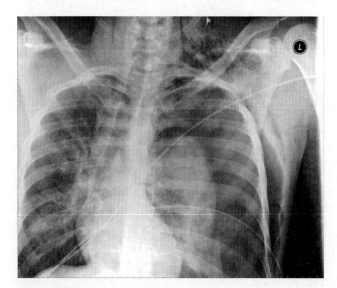

Figure 3B-6 An x-ray showing a left tension pneumothorax.

Courtesy of Dr. Mark Gestring, MD, FACS.

Signs of Tension Pneumothorax

Although the following signs are frequently discussed with a tension pneumothorax, many may not be present or are difficult to identify in the field.

Auscultation

- Decreased breath sounds on the injured side (most helpful part of physical exam)

Ultrasound

- Absence of lung sliding

Observation

- Cyanosis (may be difficult to see in the field)
- Distended neck veins (may not be present if significant blood loss)

Palpation

- Subcutaneous emphysema
- Tracheal deviation (late sign/difficult to diagnose by palpation)

FOR MORE INFORMATION

Refer to the "Pneumothorax" section of Chapter 10: Thoracic Trauma in the PHTLS 10th edition main text.

Endotracheal Intubation

Traditionally, endotracheal intubation (ETI) was considered the ideal method for achieving maximum control of the airway in trauma patients who are apneic, are unable to maintain/protect their airways, or require assisted ventilation (**Figure 3B-8**). However, its use has recently become more controversial, because in terms of patient survival, the results of using this technique have been variable.

Emergency intubation of a critical patient in the prehospital environment is a very risky procedure and has been associated with serious complications. Studies have shown that in an urban environment, critically injured trauma patients with ETI had no better outcome than those transported with a bag-mask device and an oropharyngeal airway (OPA). However, a better

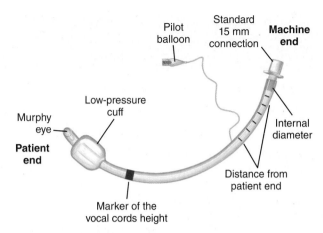

Figure 3B-8 Characteristic features of an endotracheal tube.
© National Association of Emergency Medical Technicians (NAEMT)

understanding of the indications and optimization of the technique might lead to a more positive impact on patient survival.

Advantages and Disadvantages of ETI

Advantages

- Definitive and tight seal of the airway
- Allows positive-pressure ventilation
- Optimal protection against bronchoaspiration

Disadvantages

- Time consuming
- Intravenous (IV) line, drugs, and monitoring needed (**Table 3B-1**)
- Skilled and experienced practitioner necessary
- High incidence of complications

The decision to perform ETI or to employ an alternative device should be made after a global evaluation of risk and benefit, including the probable difficulty, the practitioner's level of experience, and local protocols. Also, the risk of hypoxia from prolonged intubation attempts for a patient who has a difficult airway needs to be weighed against the need to insert the endotracheal (ET) tube in the field.

Consideration should also be given to the effect of the increase in scene time necessary to perform the procedure. For example, although there might be good reasons to intubate a patient with airway burns for a 30-minute flight to the hospital, those reasons are less compelling if the patient is unconscious and hypotensive with no facial trauma and is 5 minutes from a well-equipped and well-staffed trauma center.

Table 3B-1 Equipment and Setup for Endotracheal Intubation		
Ventilation and Oxygenation	**Intubation**	**Rescue Plan**
Bag-mask device	Endotracheal tube with cuff	Laryngeal mask
Oxygen tank	Syringe	Surgical airway set
Mask	Stylet	
Oropharyngeal airway	Laryngoscope	
Nasopharyngeal airway	Rigid, large-bore suction catheter	
Monitoring with ECG, noninvasive blood pressure, SpO$_2$, and end-tidal carbon dioxide (ETCO$_2$)		
IV access with sedative drugs, muscle relaxants, and vasopressors		

© National Association of Emergency Medical Technicians (NAEMT)

Methods of ETI

- Orotracheal intubation
- Nasotracheal intubation
- Face-to-face intubation
- Intubation with laryngeal mask
- Intubation with video laryngoscope (**Figure 3B-9**)
- Drug-assisted intubation

On the Plus Side . . .

Despite the potential challenges of this procedure, the endotracheal intubation method of airway control:

- Isolates the airway
- Allows for ventilation with 100% oxygen (fraction of inspired oxygen of 1.0)
- Eliminates the need to maintain an adequate mask-to-face seal
- Significantly decreases the risk of aspiration (vomitus, foreign material, blood)
- Facilitates deep tracheal suctioning
- Prevents gastric distention

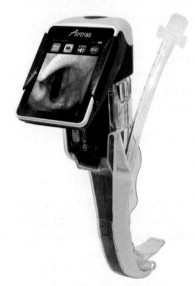

Figure 3B-9 Channeled video laryngoscope.
Courtesy of Airtaq LLC, a subsidiary of Prodol Meditec S.A.

HEAVEN Assessment for Difficult Intubation

Prior to performing an endotracheal intubation, it is imperative to perform an assessment of the intubation to be done. You will also need to take into consideration the differences in pediatric and geriatric populations that may affect airway management, which can be found in Chapter 3A.

HEAVEN is a set of criteria developed in 2015 to predict difficult intubation. These criteria seem to be better adapted to trauma patients in the prehospital environment than traditional hospital or office-based evaluation methods.

Factors That Contribute to Difficult Intubation

- Receding chin
- Short neck
- Large tongue
- Small mouth opening
- Cervical immobilization or stiff neck
- Facial trauma
- Bleeding into the airway
- Active vomiting
- Access to the patient
- Obesity

The HEAVEN criteria have been validated with peer-reviewed research and are as follows:

H—*Hypoxemia:* Oxygen saturation value ≤ 93% at the time of initial laryngoscopy

E—*Extremes of size:* Pediatric patient ≤ 8 years of age or clinical obesity

A—*Anatomic challenge:* Includes trauma, mass, swelling, foreign body, or other structural abnormality limiting laryngoscopic view

V—*Vomit/blood/fluid:* Clinically significant fluid present in the pharynx/hypopharynx at the time of laryngoscopy

E—*Exsanguination:* Suspected anemia that could potentially accelerate desaturation during rapid-sequence intubation–associated apnea

N—*Neck:* Limited cervical range of motion

FOR MORE INFORMATION

Refer to the "Endotracheal Intubation" section of Chapter 7: Airway and Ventilation in the PHTLS 10th edition main text.

CASE STUDY: DISPATCH

You are dispatched to a motorcyclist down. Patient is a 22-year-old male. It is a cool autumn day, 65°F (18°C), at approximately 1600.

Another driver witnessed the motorcyclist jerk abruptly to the right to avoid striking a large deer that ran into the roadway. The roadway is a 50 mph (80.4 kph) secondary road in a rural area. The motorcycle continued to travel off the roadway and into the woods where it struck a large downed tree and threw the rider 20 to 25 feet (6 to 7.6 meters).

First responder fire department and law enforcement officers are arriving on scene along with EMS.

A Level I trauma center is 60 minutes away by ground, 20 minutes by medevac. The local hospital emergency department is 40 minutes away by ground.

Question:

■ What injuries to the patient do you expect given the scenario?

Drug-Assisted Intubation

Drug-assisted intubation (DAI), also known as pharmacologically assisted intubation, is the use of medications to facilitate intubation. DAI increases the success rate of intubation; however, pharmacologic sedation and relaxation bring the risk of respiratory depression, apnea, and circulatory collapse. Nonetheless, in skilled hands, this technique can facilitate effective airway control when other methods fail or are otherwise not acceptable. Drug-assisted intubation can involve the use of sedation only or a combination of sedation and paralysis to prepare the patient for intubation, depending on the situation. There are three sequences of DAI:

- *Intubation using only sedatives or narcotics* may be used to relax the patient enough to permit intubation, but not prevent protective reflexes or breathing (**Figure 3B-10**).
  - Allows for the patient to be sedated and maintain muscle tone to prevent the flow of gastric contents up the esophagus and into the airway. (Loss of muscle tone can allow gastric contents to flow up the esophagus into the airway. All patients are assumed to have a full stomach.)
  - Elevating the head and thorax to 30 degrees can impede the flow of gastric contents via gravity and help protect the airway. (The head of a backboard can be elevated.)
- *Rapid-sequence intubation (RSI)* is an anesthesia technique focused on preventing aspiration and uses both sedation and paralysis medications (**Figure 3B-11**).
  - Sedation and paralysis require EMS practitioners to maintain the airway and ventilate the patient.

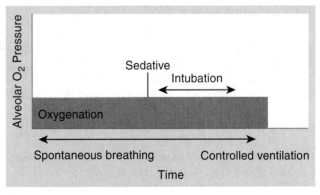

Figure 3B-10 Drug-assisted intubation. The patient is given a sedative/anesthetic to facilitate intubation. The patient continues to breathe throughout the procedure, reducing desaturation risk.

© National Association of Emergency Medical Technicians (NAEMT)

- The lack of muscle tone can lead to gastric contents flowing into the esophagus and into the airway.
- *Delayed-sequence intubation (DSI)* focuses on preventing desaturation and hypoxia. DSI is a newer technique that emphasizes preoxygenation with continuous positive-airway pressure (CPAP) and apneic oxygenation during intubation (**Figure 3B-12**).

CASE STUDY: INITIAL IMPRESSION

Law enforcement officers and the fire department are on scene—simultaneous arrival. First responder fire fighters are at the patient's side. After rolling the patient into a supine position and maintaining manual c-spine precautions, they properly remove the patient's full-face helmet. Patient is unresponsive with snoring and gurgling respirations. No serious hemorrhage is noted.

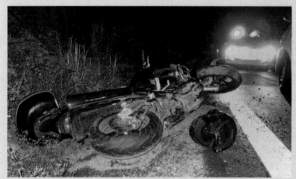

© Branislav Cerven/Shutterstock

Questions:
- What are the potential scene hazards?
- What are the potential vehicle hazards?

CASE STUDY: PRIMARY SURVEY

- **X**—No serious hemorrhage noted.
- **A**—Snoring respirations with gurgling heard in the airway; c-spine maintained manually by fire fighter first responders.
- **B**—Fast and shallow respirations; paradoxical chest movement and absent breath sounds on the right.
- **C**—Patient has a strong and regular radial pulse.
- **D**—Patient is unconscious and responsive to painful stimuli only: GCS 7 (E2, V2, M3).
- **E**—Patient is supine on the ground. Multiple small abrasions and lacerations to face and head, and upper and lower extremities; closed femur fracture.

Questions:
- What life threats need to be addressed?
- Is the patient maintaining his airway?
- Is airway and breathing management indicated?
- What areas need to be addressed before moving on with the assessment?
- What could be the cause of the breathing issue?

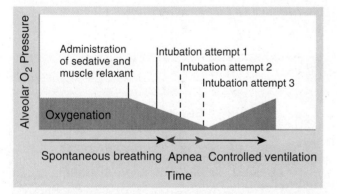

Figure 3B-11 Rapid-sequence intubation. RSI is a technique aimed at preventing bronchoaspiration. The patient is given a sedative and a rapid-acting muscle relaxant simultaneously, and then intubated. This method has a high rate of success, but there is an increased risk of hypoxia during the apnea period if the patient is not well oxygenated at the start of the procedure or if intubation attempts are prolonged.

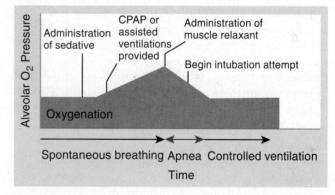

Figure 3B-12 Delayed-sequence intubation. DSI is a technique developed to reduce the risk of desaturation and hypoxia in high-risk patients. The patient is given a sedative to make preoxygenation with continuous positive airway pressure (CPAP) and/or assisted ventilations possible before the muscle relaxant is given. This method has a high rate of success and added safety, but additional time is needed to optimize preoxygenation.

CASE STUDY: DETAILED ASSESSMENT

SAMPLER assessment cannot be obtained because the patient is unconscious.

Vital Signs:

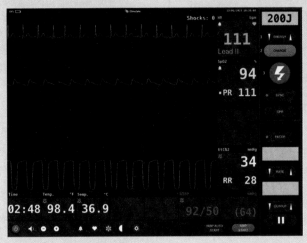

© National Association of Emergency Medical Technicians (NAEMT)

Secondary Assessment:

Detailed Physical Exam

HEENT:

(+) Airway gurgling.
PERRL
Multiple small abrasions and lacerations to face and head; no bleeding

Heart and Lungs:

Lung sounds clear on left, absent on right, shallow, fast
Heart sounds are normal, no murmur.

Neuro:

Unresponsive, except to pain
GCS 7 (E2, V2, M3)

Abdomen and Pelvis:

Soft, nontender.
Bowel sounds are normal.

Upper Extremities:

Multiple abrasions and small lacerations

Lower Extremities:

Left femur fracture evident (closed)
Multiple abrasions
Small lacerations to both legs

© National Association of Emergency Medical Technicians (NAEMT)

Primary Survey Reassessment:

- **X**—No external hemorrhage.
- **A**—Held open with a trauma jaw thrust and NPA. C-collar in place.
- **B**—NPA is in place, and patient is being ventilated with a bag-mask device at a rate of 10 to 12 bpm.
- **C**—Radial pulse is present and stronger than initial assessment findings.
- **D**—Patient remains unconscious and responsive to painful stimuli only.
- **E**—Multiple small abrasions and lacerations to face and head, and upper and lower extremities; closed femur fracture.

Question:

- When should the secondary survey be performed?

CRITICAL THINKING QUESTION

How will you prepare the patient for intubation using DAI?

- Positioning (align the axis of the airways)
- Suctioning
- Ensuring access to backup airway devices such as supraglottic airways
- Using additional devices to assist with the intubation process (bougie, video laryngoscopy)

To maximize the effectiveness of this procedure and ensure patient safety, prehospital care practitioners need to be familiar with applicable local protocols, medications, and indications for use of the technique. Drug-assisted intubation of any type requires time. Intubated patients should be sedated for transport according to local protocols. Be aware that sedation may decrease the work of breathing and any "fighting the ventilator" when mechanical ventilation is being used. If sedating the patient, small doses of benzodiazepines should be titrated intravenously. Always exercise caution whenever considering the use of medications for intubation.

Pharmacologically Assisted Intubation Indications, Contraindications, and Complications

Indications

- A patient who requires a secure airway and is difficult to intubate because of uncooperative behavior (as induced by hypoxia, traumatic brain injury, hypotension, or intoxication)

Relative Contraindications

- Availability of an alternative airway (e.g., supraglottic)
- Severe facial trauma that would impair or preclude successful intubation
- Neck deformity or swelling that complicates or precludes placement of a surgical airway
- Medical problems that would preclude use of indicated medications

Absolute Contraindications

- Known allergies to indicated medications
- Inability to intubate
- Inability to maintain airway with bag-mask device and OPA

Complications

- Inability to insert the ET tube in a sedated or paralyzed patient no longer able to protect his or her airway or breathe spontaneously; patients who are medicated and then cannot be intubated require prolonged bag-mask ventilation until the medication wears off.
- Development of hypoxia or hypercarbia during prolonged intubation attempts.
- Aspiration.
- Hypotension—virtually all of the medications have the side effect of decreasing blood pressure.

FOR MORE INFORMATION

Refer to the "Endotracheal Intubation: Drug-Assisted Intubation" section of Chapter 7: Airway and Ventilation in the PHTLS 10th edition main text.

Pulse Oximetry

Assessment of lung function can be difficult in the field, and constant ventilatory monitoring is crucial to avoid patient deterioration. Pulse oximetry and capnography are useful tools, because ventilatory rate and tidal volume can provide vital information for adjusting treatment to maintain patient oxygen levels in the field and en route.

Appropriate use of pulse oximetry devices allows early detection of pulmonary compromise or cardiovascular deterioration before physical signs are clear. Pulse oximeters are useful in prehospital applications because of their high reliability, portability, ease of application, and applicability across all age ranges and races.

Pulse oximeters provide measurements of oxygen saturation (SpO_2) and pulse rate. SpO_2 is determined by measuring the absorption ratio of red and infrared light passed through tissue. Due to the dissociation curve of hemoglobin, when SpO_2 falls below 90%, the effectiveness of oxygen delivery to the tissues can deteriorate rapidly (**Figure 3B-13**).

To ensure accurate pulse oximetry readings, follow these general guidelines:

1. Use the appropriate size and type of sensor.
2. Ensure proper alignment of sensor light.
3. Ensure that sources and photodetectors are clean, dry, and in good repair.

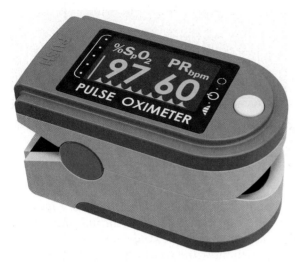

Figure 3B-13 Pulse oximetry. Most pulse oximeters will display the SpO₂ value as well as the pulse rate. It is important to realize that 90% SpO₂ is not merely 100% minus 10%; rather, it represents the flipping point beyond which desaturation progresses very quickly.

© natatravel/Shutterstock

4. Avoid sensor placement on grossly edematous (swollen) sites.
5. Remove any nail polish that may be present.
6. Limit patient movement, because excessive motion can cause inaccurate readings.

Consider the Shortfalls

Physiologic conditions that can render pulse oximetry inaccurate include:

- Shock can affect peripheral circulation through increased peripheral vascular resistance, resulting in decreased blood flow to the capillaries.
- Hypothermia can cause decreased blood flow to the periphery, resulting in decreased blood flow to the capillaries.
- Anemia can affect readings.
- Carbon monoxide and hydrogen cyanide inhalation can affect readings.

If a pulse oximeter reading does not match your patient presentation, *go with your patient presentation* and treat accordingly.

Evaluate the effectiveness of your ventilations, but good chest rise and fall, skin color improvement, mentation improvements, and most of all your patient's vital signs are important indicators.

CRITICAL THINKING QUESTIONS

Is pulse oximetry 100% accurate?

- No, it can be affected by multiple situations, particularly when using fingertip probes.

What features should the pulse oximetry have for functionality?

- Pulse rate display, SpO₂ display, and waveform display

Capnography

Capnography, or end-tidal carbon dioxide ($ETCO_2$) monitoring, has been used in critical care units for many years. Recent advances in technology have allowed smaller, more durable units to be produced for prehospital use. Detecting CO_2 in expired air confirms that the patient has an active metabolism that is able to generate CO_2 as a byproduct of that metabolism. In addition, the presence of CO_2 in expired air confirms that there is sufficient ongoing circulation to bring CO_2 to the lungs and that effective alveolar ventilation and air exchange are taking place. Continuous capnography provides another tool and must be correlated with all other information about a patient.

This technique places a sensor directly into the "mainstream" of the exhaled gas. In a patient being ventilated with a bag-mask device, the sensor is placed between the bag-mask device and the ET tube. A normal $ETCO_2$ reading is between 30 and 40 mm Hg; working to maintain readings within normal ranges will usually be beneficial to the patient.

Figure 3B-14 shows a normal end-tidal waveform, and **Figure 3B-15** illustrates the different phases of the respiratory cycle. These can be useful when comparing to an $ETCO_2$ reading in a critical trauma patient.

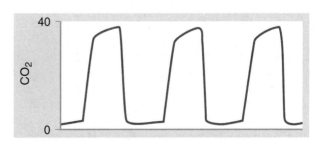

Figure 3B-14 Normal end-tidal capnography waveform.

© plo/Shutterstock

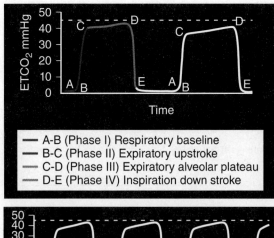

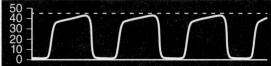

Figure 3B-15 The graph (waveform) shows how much CO_2 is present in each phase of the respiratory cycle: Phase I: Respiratory baseline; Phase II: expiratory upstroke; Phase III: Expiratory alveolar plateau; Phase IV: inspiration downstroke.

© Jones & Bartlett Learning

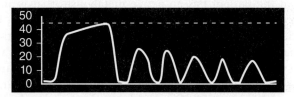

Figure 3B-16 Capnography waveform trending down in shock.

© Jones & Bartlett Learning

Capnography is the gold standard for monitoring proper ET tube placement; a sudden drop in expired carbon dioxide, as may result either from dislodgement of the ET tube or from decreased perfusion, should prompt a reevaluation of patient status and ET tube position. Monitoring closely for changes can indicate when the patient is deteriorating.

Know When to Monitor

Initial transport decisions are based on clinical findings; for example, it would be inappropriate to take time at the scene to place the patient on monitors if the patient is losing blood. Instead, capnography should be applied en route to the hospital.

Consider the following examples. **Figure 3B-16** is a capnography waveform trending down in shock. The waveform shows decreased to no metabolism due to

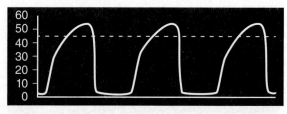

Figure 3B-17 Capnography waveform indicating hypoxia due to asthma.

© Jones & Bartlett Learning

death of the cells, and subsequently tissue. **Figure 3B-17** shows the capnography waveform indicating hypoxia due to asthma. The waveform shows bronchoconstriction in a patient with bronchospasm.

QUICK TIP

$ETCO_2$ is the ultimate means to determine that air exchange is taking place. It is standard practice in EMS to have a working CO_2 monitor when employing an advanced airway management technique.

QUICK TIP

In a pediatric patient, use a properly fitted oxygen mask and the "squeeze-release-release" timing technique. Watch for rise and fall of the chest, and if $ETCO_2$ monitoring is available, maintain levels between 35 and 40 mm Hg.

Surgical Airway

Surgical cricothyrotomy is a type of definitive airway that involves the creation of a surgical opening in the cricothyroid membrane, which lies between the larynx (thyroid cartilage) and the cricoid cartilage, through which a tube is directed into the tracheal lumen (**Figure 3B-18**). In most patients, the skin is very thin in this location, making it amenable to immediate access to the airway.

The use of this surgical airway in the prehospital arena is controversial. Complications are common with this procedure, it requires frequent practice on real tissue as well as a high skill level, and there is no second chance to get it right.

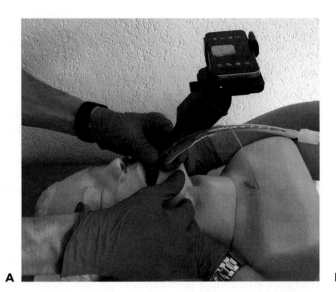

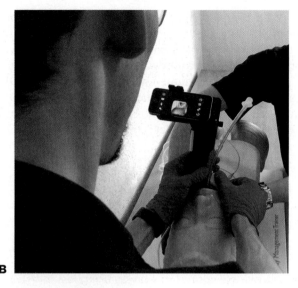

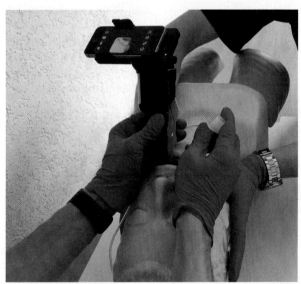

Figure 3B-18 Surgical cricothyrotomy. **A.** The left hand executes the "laryngeal handshake," with both the thumb and middle finger stabilizing the larynx while the index finger locates the cricothyroid membrane. The palm of the hand will help to keep the chin out of the way. **B.** A 2- to 3-cm vertical incision is made over the cricothyroid cartilage down to the cricoid, and the membrane is located by palpation with the index finger. **C.** A hook is introduced into the incision and is lifted upward, providing an opening directed toward the trachea. The tube is introduced into the trachea, and the cuff is inflated.

© Jones & Bartlett Learning. Photographed by Glen Ellman.

CRITICAL THINKING QUESTION

What complications are common with surgical cricothyrotomy?

- Prolonged procedure time
- Hemorrhage
- Aspiration
- Misplacement or false passage of the ET tube
- Injury to neck structures or vessels
- Perforation of the esophagus

Keep Away from Children

Surgical cricothyrotomy is contraindicated in the care of a pediatric trauma patient. This technique is not recommended in children younger than 10 years because the very soft cartilage makes incision difficult and the thick mucosa under the glottis makes it very difficult to find the lumen.

With complex skills such as intubation or surgical cricothyrotomy, the more times a skill is performed, the better the chance for a successful outcome. However, for surgical cricothyrotomy, taking the time to practice or train for this technique must be weighed against the potential benefit of using that time to train in ETI, because proficient ETI skills should dramatically minimize the need to even consider surgical cricothyrotomy for most patients.

Indications and Contraindications for Surgical Cricothyrotomy

Indications

- Massive midface and/or oral trauma precluding the use of a bag-mask device
- Inability to control the airway using less invasive maneuvers

Contraindications

- Any patient who can be safely intubated, either orally or nasally
- Patients with laryngotracheal injuries
- Children under 10 years of age
- Patients with acute laryngeal disease of traumatic or infectious origin
- Insufficient training

CASE STUDY: ONGOING MANAGEMENT

The patient remains unconscious and is unable to support his airway.

Questions:

- Is the patient stable or unstable?
- How will you manage the patient?
- What is your continued airway assessment plan?
- How will you assess the adequacy of the patient's airway and breathing?
- Would a supraglottic airway be considered in this situation?
- Is this patient a candidate for DAI?

Prolonged Transport

Airway management of a patient prior to and during a prolonged transport requires complex decision making. Interventions to control and secure the airway, especially using complex techniques, depend on a number of factors, including:

- The patient's injuries
- The clinical skills of the practitioner
- The equipment available
- The distance and transport time to definitive care

Consider the risks and benefits of all the airway options available before making a final airway decision. Both a longer distance of transport and a longer transport time lower the threshold for securing the airway with endotracheal intubation. For transports of 15 to 20 minutes, essential skills, including an oral airway and bag-mask ventilation, may be sufficient. Use of air medical transport also lowers the threshold to perform endotracheal intubation, because a cramped, noisy environment makes ongoing airway assessment and management difficult.

Continuous pulse oximetry monitoring should be used for all trauma patients during transport, and capnography should be considered mandatory for all intubated patients. Confirmation of ETI should be performed each time the patient is moved or repositioned. Prior to a prolonged transport, potential oxygen needs should be calculated and made available for the transport. The patient should be maintained on the lowest inspired oxygen concentration that assures a saturation > 94%. Intubated patients should be sedated for the transport according to local protocols.

FOR MORE INFORMATION

Refer to the "Surgical Airway" section of Chapter 7: Airway and Ventilation in the PHTLS 10th edition main text.

Don't Be a Dope! Use the DOPE Mnemonic!

A change in an intubated patient's status requires immediate reassessment.

Use the DOPE mnemonic:

- **D**—*Dislodgement/Displacement:* Reassess at the ET tube depth from the initial depth during intubation and adjust the ET tube if needed.
- **O**—*Obstruction:* Reassess breath sounds and suction the ET tube if needed.
- **P**—*Pneumothorax:* Rule out pneumothorax by assessing both lung fields.
- **E**—*Equipment:* Check equipment, and swap out if an equipment issue is discovered. If using a ventilator, switch to a bag-mask device and check lung compliance with the bag.

Complete a primary survey.

- Because there has been a change in status, a primary survey should be repeated to address life threats in addition to the DOPE assessment.

You frequently reassess the patient during transport to be sure the monitor matches the patient's current clinical condition.

Questions:

- What type of facility are you transporting your patient to?
- What are the pros and cons of ETCO$_2$ and SpO$_2$ monitoring?
- What should you do if there is inconsistent data from electronic monitoring devices that does not match the patient's current clinical condition?

It was decided to transport to a Level I trauma center via medevac. The patient was placed on a backboard, secured, covered with a blanket for warmth, and moved to a Stokes basket to be carried out of the woods and brush over the rough terrain.

The patient had surgery to correct the hemopneumothorax and the fractured femur. The patient was intubated, and subsequently a tracheostomy was performed.

The patient died one week later in the surgical intensive care unit due to severe chest trauma.

FOR MORE INFORMATION

Refer to the "Prolonged Transport" section of Chapter 7: Airway and Ventilation in the PHTLS 10th edition main text.

SUMMARY

- In the prehospital setting, maintaining adequate tidal volume is the primary concern in trauma patients.

- Pulse oximetry is a useful tool; however, many conditions can render the results useless. If a pulse oximeter reading does not match your patient presentation, go with your patient presentation and treat accordingly.

- In capnography, end-tidal carbon dioxide (ETCO$_2$) assists with assessment of a patient's ventilatory status and is a reliable and very sensitive indicator of ongoing air exchange and circulation.

- Thoracic trauma often impacts the proper functioning of the respiratory system. When present, assess the patient for airway and breathing issues and treat accordingly.

- Endotracheal intubation is controversial, especially in the field. Know your limitations. If you know that intubation is not your strength, allow a more experienced practitioner to perform it.

- A solid knowledge base of medications is necessary to perform drug-assisted intubation.

- The use of surgical cricothyrotomy in the prehospital arena is controversial because there are many complications and contraindications. Only the most experienced practitioners may perform this surgical airway within local protocols.

- Both a longer distance of transport and a longer transport time lower the threshold for securing the airway with endotracheal intubation, as does air medical transport. Prior to a prolonged transport, potential oxygen needs should be calculated and made available for the transport.

CASE STUDY RECAP

Dispatch

What injuries to the patient do you expect given the scenario?	<ul><li>Airway obstruction</li><li>Brain injury</li><li>Spine injury</li><li>Thoracic trauma—possible flail chest and/or pneumothorax</li><li>Hemorrhage—internal and external</li><li>Fractures</li></ul>

Initial Impression

What are the potential scene hazards?	<ul><li>Uneven terrain</li><li>Long distance off the roadway to less stable ground</li><li>Obstacles to scale going into where the patient is or moving the patient out (e.g., downed tree)</li></ul>
What may be potential vehicle hazards?	<ul><li>Electrical shorts</li><li>Fire</li><li>Fuel and other fluid leaks</li></ul>

Primary Survey

What life threats need to be addressed?	<ul><li>Airway compromise</li><li>Breathing rate and depth compromised</li><li>Patient being unconscious and responsive to pain only</li></ul>
Is the patient maintaining his airway?	<ul><li>No. The airway is not patent. It needs to be repositioned, suctioned, and an airway adjunct placed.</li></ul>
Is airway and breathing management indicated?	<ul><li>Yes. Reposition and open the airway with a trauma jaw thrust, place a basic airway adjunct, and ventilate with a bag-valve mask to support ventilations.</li><li>Needle chest decompression for tension pneumothorax.</li></ul>
What areas need to be addressed before moving on with the assessment?	<ul><li>Airway management including ventilations with a bag-valve mask and airway adjunct. Needle chest decompression.</li></ul>
What could be the cause of the breathing issue?	<ul><li>Chest trauma including pneumothorax, tension pneumothorax, hemothorax, fractured ribs, and diaphragm injury.</li></ul>

Detailed Assessment

When should the secondary survey be performed?	<ul><li>Secondary survey may be delayed due to the presence of life threats and associated treatment.</li><li>If other EMS personnel are present, secondary and vitals may be performed simultaneously with management of the life threats.</li></ul>

Ongoing Management

Is the patient stable or unstable?	<ul><li>Patient is unstable but can be stabilized based on airway and ventilation management choices.</li></ul>
How will you manage the patient?	<ul><li>Treat immediate life threats.</li><li>Reassess the life threat management, spinal stabilization, airway management, choose the appropriate destination and transport method, and package for transport.</li></ul>

What is your continued airway assessment plan?	■ Assess for effectiveness of current interventions. ■ Suction as needed to manage blood or secretions in the airway.
How will you assess the adequacy of the patient's airway and breathing?	■ Assess the adequacy of bag-mask ventilations, pulse oximetry, $ETCO_2$ reading, lung sounds, and chest rise symmetry.
Would a supraglottic airway work in this situation?	■ A supraglottic airway is contraindicated in a patient with the ability to swallow. Endotracheal intubation with DAI/RSI could be considered for this patient. This is a time-consuming procedure, and the proximity to the trauma center as well as whether bag-mask ventilations with basic airway adjunct are effective should be considered.
Is the patient a candidate for DAI?	■ Yes. Due to the proximity to a Level I trauma center, medevac availability, and the patient's anticipated clinical course and ability to maintain a patent airway, this should be considered.
Transport	
What type of facility are you transporting your patient to?	■ Level I trauma center due to significant head injury and airway compromise. Neurosurgery capabilities are necessary.
How can you accomplish $ETCO_2$ and SpO_2 monitoring?	■ Waveform capnography is the ideal method for $ETCO_2$. (Normal values are 35–45%.) ■ Pulse oximetry with waveform is the ideal method for SpO_2. (94% or above is optimal.)
What should you do if there is inconsistent data from electronic monitoring devices that do not match the patient's current clinical condition?	■ If there are inconsistent data from electronic monitoring devices, reassess to be sure the monitor matches the patient's current clinical condition. ■ Treat the patient, not the monitor.

STUDY QUESTIONS

1. You have been performing ongoing management on a 35-year-old female patient who sustained thoracic trauma when a car hit her as she crossed the street. Originally, your electronic monitoring devices all produce results consistent with your patient's clinical condition. However, en route to the trauma center, the monitors start to differ from your patient's current clinical condition each time you reassess. How should you handle this situation?
   A. Treat the patient's condition, not the monitor results.
   B. Continue to reassess the patient and record the results for the trauma center.
   C. Treat your patient based on the test results.
   D. Stop testing and wait until you arrive at the trauma center for them to perform an assessment.

2. You have determined that you are going to need to perform orotracheal intubation on a 50-year-old male motor vehicle crash (MVC) critically injured trauma patient due to prolonged transport time. What do you need to do first?
   A. Preoxygenate to maximize oxygen saturation.
   B. Place the patient in a "sniffing" position.
   C. Clear the mouth of any obstructions.
   D. Prepare the patient for immediate transport.

3. You are oxygenating a pediatric patient using a properly fitted oxygen mask and the "squeeze-release-release" timing technique. As you watch for the rise and fall of the chest, you check end-tidal CO_2 ($ETCO_2$) monitoring aiming to maintain what level?
   A. Between 40 and 45 mm Hg
   B. Between 30 and 35 mm Hg
   C. Between 35 and 40 mm Hg
   D. The level is irrelevant because capnography is inaccurate in pediatric patients.

4. What is one reason to use capnography as part of your patient reassessment?
   A. To get accurate readings for blood pressure
   B. To assure proper ET tube placement
   C. To measure arterial blood saturation
   D. To ensure proper placement for needle decompression

ANSWER KEY

Question 1: A
If there are inconsistent data from electronic monitoring devices, reassess to be sure the monitor matches the patient's current clinical condition. However, it is most important to treat the patient, not the monitor, so use other signs and symptoms of potential patient deterioration.

Question 2: A
Before insertion of any invasive airway, the patient is preoxygenated with a high concentration of oxygen using a simple airway adjunct or manual airway procedure.

Question 3: C
The proper level to maintain is between 35 and 40 mm Hg.

Question 4: B
Capnography can monitor proper endotracheal tube placement. It doesn't read blood pressure, so it cannot be used to determine if a patient is hypotensive. Pulse oximetry, not capnography, measures arterial blood saturation. Capnography is not useful in needle decompression.

REFERENCES AND FURTHER READING

Crewdson K, Lockey DJ, Røislien J, Lossius HM, Rehn M. The success of pre-hospital tracheal intubation by different pre-hospital providers: a systematic literature review and meta-analysis. *Critical Care.* 2017;21(31). https://ccforum.biomedcentral.com/articles/10.1186/s13054-017-1603-7. Accessed November 15, 2018.

Davis D, Olvera DJ. HEAVEN criteria: derivation of a new difficult airway prediction tool. *Air Med J.* 2017;36(4): 195-197. https://doi.org/10.1016/j.amj.2017.04.001

Moy HP. Evidence-based EMS: endotracheal intubation. *EMS World.* 2015;44(1):30-32, 34. https://www.emsworld.com/article/206057/evidence-based-ems-endotracheal-intubation. Accessed November 15, 2018.

National Association of Emergency Medical Technicians. *PHTLS: Prehospital Trauma Life Support.* 10th ed. Burlington, MA: Public Safety Group; 2023.

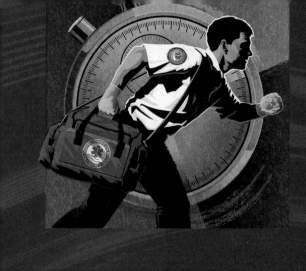

CHAPTER 4

C—Circulation

LESSON OBJECTIVES

· Describe the pathophysiology of shock.
· Recognize the clinical signs of shock.
· Explain the assessment and management of a patient experiencing shock.
· Identify the modalities of fluid resuscitation.
· Recognize additional hemorrhagic shock management strategies, such as blood component therapy and transexamic acid (TXA).
· Describe special considerations in shock management.

Introduction

A major complication of disrupting the normal physiology of life is known as *shock*. Shock results from a lack of oxygen perfusing to the tissues. It is a highly time-sensitive issue because our bodies have no real oxygen reserves—we have fat stores for 30 days and glucose stores for 1 day, but we have only enough oxygen reserves for about 5 minutes. If oxygen supply to the tissues is interrupted, organ damage sets in within minutes and, at a certain point, becomes irreversible. Shock is truly "death in progress," so urgent intervention is needed.

Definition of Shock

Shock is defined as inadequate cellular perfusion. Cells require oxygen and glucose to produce energy (adenosine triphosphate [ATP]). Oxygen in the blood can only be transported when it is bound to hemoglobin (Hb) in red blood cells (RBCs), and one molecule of Hb can only transport four molecules of oxygen. Low oxygen content in the blood is known as *hypoxemia*. Hypoxemia leads to *hypoxia*, which occurs when the oxygen content of the body's tissues and cells is low. Finally, insufficient blood flow cannot provide oxygen to the cells, which is known as *ischemia*. Ischemic sensitivity varies by organ (e.g., the brain, lungs, and heart have the greatest ischemic sensitivity).

The only way for the body to transport more oxygen is to speed up the circulation of RBCs—that is, to make the heart beat faster. If the number of circulating RBCs decreases, so does oxygen transport capacity. At some point, the remaining blood will not be able to circulate fast enough, the tissues will not get enough oxygen, and the body is then in shock.

CASE STUDY: **DISPATCH**

You are dispatched at 1300 to the scene of a motorcycle collision on a rural roadway. The patient is a 29-year-old male. The speed limit is 55 mph (88 kph), but the speed of the driver when the collision occurred is unknown. He veered off the road, rolling several times before impact into a telephone pole.

The patient was found lying supine on the ground approximately 50 feet (15.2 m) from the point of impact. It is a sunny, cool, fall day with a temperature of 50°F (10°C).

Question:

■ What potential injuries do you expect this patient to have based on the available information?

Cellular Physiology

- Cellular perfusion comes from sufficient blood flow and oxygen.
- Aerobic metabolism produces sufficient energy for cellular functions.
  - Aerobic metabolism of glucose with oxygen produces 38 ATP molecules.
- Waste products from aerobic metabolism are CO_2 and H_2O.

Every Blood Cell Counts

There are three components necessary for oxygenation of the cells in the body (also known as the Fick principle):

- On-loading of oxygen to RBCs in the lung
- Delivery of RBCs to tissue cells
- Off-loading of oxygen from RBCs to tissue cells

A crucial part of this process is that the patient must have enough RBCs available to deliver adequate amounts of oxygen to tissue cells in order to produce energy.

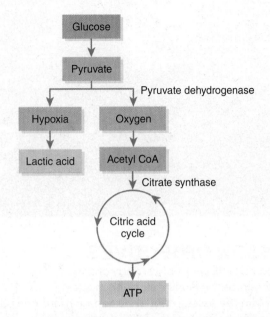

Figure 4-1 The formation of lactate during hypoxia. In the face of hypoxia, pyruvate is converted to lactic acid rather than being processed by the citric acid cycle to make adenosine triphosphate (ATP).

© National Association of Emergency Medical Technicians (NAEMT)

Table 4-1 Organ Tolerance to Ischemia	
Organ	**Ischemic Sensitivity Time**
Heart, brain, lungs	4 to 6 minutes
Kidneys, liver, gastrointestinal tract	45 to 90 minutes
Muscle, bone, skin	4 to 6 hours

Modified from American College of Surgeons Committee on Trauma. *Advanced Trauma Life Support for Doctors: Student Course Manual.* 7th ed. American College of Surgeons; 2004.

Pathophysiology of Shock

Cells maintain their normal metabolic functions by producing and using energy in the form of ATP. The most efficient method of generating energy is through aerobic metabolism. The cells take in oxygen and glucose and metabolize them through a complicated process that produces energy, along with the by-products of water and carbon dioxide.

Anaerobic metabolism, in contrast, occurs without the use of oxygen. It is the backup power system in the body and uses stored body fat as its energy source. However, anaerobic metabolism is not an ideal source of energy, because it:

- Can run only for a short time
- Produces 19 times less energy than aerobic metabolism
  - Aerobic metabolism of glucose with oxygen produces 38 ATP molecules, along with carbon dioxide and water as waste products.
  - Anaerobic metabolism produces 2 ATP molecules per glucose molecule, along with lactic acid as a waste product (**Figure 4-1**).
  - Lactic acid accumulation results in metabolic acidosis.
- May ultimately become irreversible

If anaerobic metabolism is not corrected quickly, cells start to die, leading to a catastrophic cascade effect. The sensitivity of cells to the lack of oxygen varies from organ system to organ system (**Table 4-1**), and it is greatest in the brain, heart, and lungs, which have about 4 to 6 minutes before irreversible damage occurs.

The Ominous Lactic Acid

In anaerobic metabolism, cells suffering from hypoxia (lack of oxygen) release lactic acid, causing acidosis and respiration increases to "blow off" the acid load. Patients in shock tend to breathe faster, even in the face of perfect lung function.

Although not toxic by itself, the accumulation of lactate in the blood is a sure sign that tissues are on an anaerobic diet and that organs are now living on borrowed time.

Causes of Altered Mental Status

The brain is sensitive to both the lack of oxygen and the effects of lactic acidosis, in addition to falling ATP levels.

Any pulse oximeter reading below 94% (at sea level) is worrisome and should serve as a stimulus to identify the cause of hypoxia.

QUICK TIP

When anaerobic metabolism kicks in, the brain's sensing system detects the abnormal increase in the amount of carbon dioxide, and it stimulates the respiratory center to increase the rate and depth of ventilation to remove the carbon dioxide. *Tachypnea* is frequently one of the earliest signs of anaerobic metabolism and shock—even earlier than increased pulse rate.

When the body is in a shock state, it diverts blood flow to save essential organs. That is why less-essential organs that still have a high oxygen need—like the kidneys, liver, lungs, bowel, and vascular endothelium—show damage first, whereas the heart and brain will be spared to the very end. Anything that negatively impacts blood circulation decreases oxygen transport to the tissues and can cause shock. Cardiogenic shock, in which the heart cannot pump adequately, or distributive shock, where dilation of the vessels diminishes venous return to the heart, are possible causes in trauma patients; however, the most frequent cause is hemorrhagic shock, resulting from the loss of circulating blood and decrease in fluid volume.

Shock Kills

Complications of shock include:

- *Vascular endothelium damage:* Results in capillary leakage and coagulopathy—onset is in the span of a few minutes
- *Renal failure:* Acute tubular necrosis and anuria—becomes manifest after 6–12 hours
- *Bowel ischemia:* Onset is within several hours, with bacterial translocation and bowel perforation
- *Shock lung:* Occurs within hours, leading to respiratory distress
- *Hepatic failure:* With coagulopathy, sepsis, multiorgan failure, and death

Transport Early

Emergency medical services (EMS) practitioners have limited means for treating blood loss and shock in the field; thus, rapid transportation to definitive care must be considered early.

FOR MORE INFORMATION

Refer to the "Physiology of Shock" section of Chapter 3: Shock: Pathophysiology of Life and Death in the PHTLS 10th edition main text.

Types of Traumatic Shock

Traumatic shock in the emergent phase involves a disruption of the cardiovascular system in one of its components: blood (fluid; hypovolemic shock), heart (pump; cardiogenic shock), and/or blood vessels (container; distributive shock). In trauma patients, hypovolemic shock as a result of blood loss (hemorrhagic shock) is the most common. **Table 4-2** lists the types of shock, and **Table 4-3** indicates the signs associated with each type.

QUICK TIP

When in doubt, always consider hypovolemic shock as the cause, because there is always some degree of hemorrhage in trauma patients.

Table 4-2 Types of Traumatic Shock

	Hypovolemic Shock	Distributive Shock (Neurogenic Hypotension)	Cardiogenic Shock
Defined as	Acute blood or fluid loss (loss of circulating volume)	Neurogenic loss of vascular tone (abnormal dilation of the vascular compartment)	Low cardiac output (impaired cardiac function)
Causes	Uncontrolled external/internal hemorrhage resulting in the loss of blood (fluid) Severe dehydration	Spinal injuries resulting in vasodilation by loss of neurogenic vascular smooth muscle tone (container)	Conditions that reduce cardiac output (pump)
Examples	Blood loss (hemorrhagic shock) Plasma loss (burn patients)	High spinal cord injury	Intrinsic: Cardiac contusion (heart muscle damage) Valvular disruption (regurgitation) Extrinsic: Cardiac tamponade (**Figure 4-2**) Tension pneumothorax (**Figure 4-3**)
Correction (can slow progression of shock and death)	Control external hemorrhage and protect the development of internal clotting (hemorrhagic) Administer fluids (nonhemorrhagic)	Increase fluid volume and promote vasoconstriction	Resolve the cause (intrinsic: supportive; extrinsic: needle decompression, pericardiocentesis)

© National Association of Emergency Medical Technicians (NAEMT)

Table 4-3 Signs Associated with Types of Shock

Vital Sign	Hypovolemic	Distributive (Neurogenic Hypotension)	Cardiogenic
Skin temperature/quality	Cool, clammy	Warm, dry	Cool, clammy
Skin color	Pale, cyanotic	Flushed	Pale, cyanotic
Blood pressure	Drops	Drops	Drops
Level of consciousness	Altered	Lucid	Altered
Capillary refill time	Slowed	Normal	Slowed

© National Association of Emergency Medical Technicians (NAEMT)

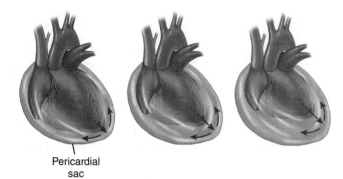

Figure 4-2 Cardiac tamponade. As blood courses from a hole in the heart muscle into the pericardial space, it limits expansion of the ventricle. Therefore, the ventricle cannot fill completely. As more blood accumulates in the pericardial space, less ventricular space is available, and cardiac output is reduced.

© National Association of Emergency Medical Technicians (NAEMT)

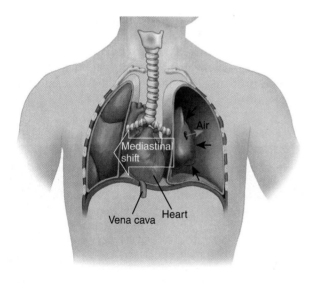

Figure 4-3 Tension pneumothorax. If the amount of air trapped in the pleural space continues to increase, not only does the lung on the affected side collapse, but the mediastinum shifts to the opposite side. The mediastinal shift impairs blood return to the heart through the venae cavae, thus affecting cardiac output, while at the same time compressing the opposite lung.

© National Association of Emergency Medical Technicians (NAEMT)

Shock and Skin/Buccal Color

- Normal skin or buccal mucosa color generally indicates a well-oxygenated patient without anaerobic metabolism.
- Cyanotic or mottled skin or mucosa indicates unoxygenated hemoglobin and a lack of adequate oxygenation to the periphery.

- Pale, mottled, or cyanotic skin/buccal mucosa has inadequate blood flow resulting from one of the following:
  - Peripheral vasoconstriction (most often associated with hypovolemia)
  - Decreased supply of RBCs (acute anemia)
  - Interruption of blood supply to that portion of the body, such as might be found with a fracture or injury of a blood vessel

---

CASE STUDY: INITIAL IMPRESSION

The motorcycle is lying adjacent to a telephone pole. There is moderate deformity to the motorcycle wheels and handlebars. The patient is found lying supine on the ground 50 feet (15.2 m) from the point of impact. An emergency vehicle is positioned at the scene to protect the scene and ensure egress of ambulance.

Question:
- What are the scene safety concerns?

Physiological Response to Shock

The body has several compensatory mechanisms that occur in response to shock:

- Cardiovascular response increases blood pressure and cardiac output. Heart rate is increased, as is the strength of contractions.
- Hemodynamic response increases blood pressure. Vasoconstriction and splenic contraction occur.
- Endocrine response supports the cardiovascular and hemodynamic compensation by the secretion of epinephrine and norepinephrine (adrenal). The sympathetic nervous system releases catecholamines. The endocrine response also engages renal compensation of sodium and fluid reabsorption through the secretion of antidiuretic hormone (posterior pituitary) and aldosterone (adrenal).
- Cellular response is energy production via anaerobic metabolism as a reaction to hypoxia.

Classes of Hemorrhage

Hemorrhagic shock is by far the most frequent cause of shock. A 150-pound (70-kg) adult human has approximately 5 liters of circulating blood volume.

Hemorrhagic shock (hypovolemic shock resulting from blood loss) is categorized into four classes, depending on the severity and amount of blood loss (**Figure 4-4**; see **Table 4-4** at the end of this section).

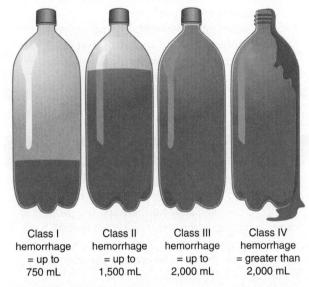

| Class I hemorrhage = up to 750 mL | Class II hemorrhage = up to 1,500 mL | Class III hemorrhage = up to 2,000 mL | Class IV hemorrhage = greater than 2,000 mL |

Figure 4-4 The approximate amount of blood loss for Class I, II, III, and IV hemorrhages.

© National Association of Emergency Medical Technicians (NAEMT)

Class I Hemorrhage

Class I hemorrhage is compensated shock, because the body can compensate for the lack of oxygen by increasing the heart rate and vascular tone (vasoconstriction). The spleen can compensate for blood loss by contracting and increasing blood volume up to 500 mL. At the time of a traumatic injury with hemorrhage, physiological signs are within normal baseline for the patient. The patient is still conscious, the skin is being perfused, urine output is normal, and the ventilatory rate is normal because there is no anaerobic metabolism to create lactic acid in the blood. The release of adrenaline is the cause of the patient being slightly anxious.

Physiological Signs: Initial Injury with Hemorrhage

- Mentation: Slightly anxious
- Skin: Warm, dry; capillary refill < 2 seconds
- Breathing: Normal rate and depth (12 to 16 breaths/minute for adults)
- Heart rate: Normal/slightly increased rate
- Pulse: Equal central and peripheral pulse strength
- Blood pressure: Normal systolic/diastolic and pulse pressure

Table 4-4 Classification of Hemorrhage				
	Class I	**Class II**	**Class III**	**Class IV**
Blood loss (mL)	< 750	750–1,500	1,500–2,000	> 2,000
Blood loss (% blood volume)	< 15%	15–30%	30–40%	> 40%
Pulse rate	↔	↔/↑	↑	↑/↑↑
Blood pressure	↔	↔	↔/↓	↓
Pulse pressure (mm Hg)	↔	↓	↓	↓
Ventilatory rate	14–20	20–30	30–40	> 35
Central nervous system/ mental status	Slightly anxious	Mildly anxious	Anxious, confused	Confused, lethargic
Base excess	0 to –2	–2 to –6	–6 to –10	More than –10
Need for blood	Monitor	Possible	Yes	Massive transfusion

↑ = increased, ↓ = decreased, ↔ = normal range

Note: The values and descriptions for the criteria listed for these classes of shock should not be interpreted as absolute determinants of the class of shock, because significant overlap exists.

Data from American College of Surgeons Committee on Trauma. *Advanced Trauma Life Support for Doctors: Student Course Manual.* 8th ed. American College of Surgeons; 2008.

Class II Hemorrhage

Class II hemorrhage may result in postural hypotension (i.e., systolic pressure drops when moving from supine to sitting/standing). As hemorrhage continues, the endocrine response from the sympathetic nervous system (secretion of epinephrine and norepinephrine) results in compensation for blood loss by vasoconstriction and increased heart rate and strength of ventricular contraction. Decreased pulse pressure is the result.

Physiological Signs: Compensation

- Mentation: Increasing anxiety, irritability, restlessness (catecholamine release)
- Skin: Pale, cool; capillary refill 2 to 3 seconds (peripheral vasoconstriction from catecholamine release)
- Breathing: Increased rate (14 to 20 breaths/minute in adults) (hypoxia)
- Heart rate: Increasing rate
- Pulse: Normal central pulses; weak peripheral pulses (catecholamine release)
- Blood pressure: Normal systolic/diastolic; decreased pulse pressure (compensation effects)

Class III Hemorrhage

Class III hemorrhage is progressing shock. If it is not reversed, it will result in multiple organ system failure, and the patient will die. As hemorrhage continues, the endocrine response continues with vasoconstriction and increased heart rate and strength of ventricular contraction; however, the compensatory mechanisms are beginning to fail with a decrease in cardiac output. Decreased blood pressure is a late sign. Increasing ventilatory rate is a compensatory mechanism to reverse the effects of lactic acidosis.

Physiological Signs: Progressing Shock

- Mentation: Increasing anxiety, irritability, and restlessness; confusion
- Skin: Pale, cool, and diaphoretic; capillary refill 3 to 4 seconds
- Breathing: Increasing rate and depth (30 to 40 breaths/minute in adults)
- Heart rate: Increasing rate
- Pulse: Weak central pulses, absent peripheral pulses
- Blood pressure: Decreasing systolic/diastolic; decreasing pulse pressure

Class IV Hemorrhage

Class IV hemorrhage is a stage of severe shock characterized by marked tachycardia (heart rate greater than 120 to 140 beats/minute), tachypnea (ventilatory rate greater than 35 breaths/minute), profound confusion or lethargy—which means that even the brain is not getting enough oxygen—and greatly decreased systolic blood pressure, typically in the range of 60 mm Hg.

Significant internal hemorrhage can occur with fractures. Fractures of the femur and pelvis are of greatest concern. A single fracture of the femur may be associated with up to 2 to 4 units (1,000 to 2,000 mL) of blood loss into a thigh. This injury alone could potentially result in the loss of 30% to 40% of an adult's blood volume, resulting in decompensated hypovolemic shock. The point of decompensation is hypotension, and death is impending.

Physiological Signs: Decompensation

- Mentation: Difficult to arouse, progressing to unresponsive
- Skin: Pale, cool, diaphoretic; capillary refill > 5 seconds
- Breathing: Increasing rate
- Heart rate: Increasing rate
- Pulse: Weak central pulses, absent peripheral pulses
- Blood pressure: Decreasing systolic/diastolic; decreasing pulse pressure

---

CASE STUDY: PRIMARY SURVEY

- **X**—No major external hemorrhage noted
- **A**—Patent
- **B**—29 breaths/minute, shallow chest rise
- **C**—Rapid, thready radial pulse; skin pale
- **D**—GCS 14 (E4, V4, M6), PERRL
- **E**—Lying supine on ground; pelvis tender to palpation; abrasion and bruising noted to left upper quadrant (LUQ), arms, and hands

Questions:

- What are the potential life threats given the mechanism of injury and primary survey results?
- Why is it important to check the airway and breathing in this patient?
- Which organ(s) in the LUQ could cause severe internal bleeding?

Special Considerations for Blood Loss

Numerous factors can complicate the assessment of the trauma patient, hiding or blunting the usual signs of shock. These factors may mislead the unwary prehospital care practitioner into thinking a trauma patient is

Table 4-5 Some Medications to Know When Treating Shock

Drug Class	Effect
Beta blockers	Prevent compensatory tachycardia and increase in cardiac output. Interfere with compensatory mechanisms and make evaluation difficult
Antihypertensive drugs	Interfere with compensatory vasoconstriction
Diuretics	Diminish circulating volume, so the patient may often be hypovolemic to begin with
Anticoagulants	Impair function of coagulation factors, so administration of factors will be necessary
Antiaggregants	Render platelets ineffective, so platelet transfusion will be needed

© National Association of Emergency Medical Technicians (NAEMT)

stable when that is not the case. Keep the following in mind:

- *Medications:* Beta blockers affect heart rate; thus, heart rate may not be able to compensate for blood loss. Platelet inactivators and anticoagulants affect clotting time (**Table 4-5**).
- *Pacemaker implants:* Fixed rate pacemakers can affect heart rate; thus, tachycardia may not be observed.
- *Geriatric/older adult patients:* Geriatric patients often take medications like beta blockers or have pacemakers, so compensatory tachycardia will be limited or even absent. In addition, a blood pressure within normal range might be hypotensive for a patient whose baseline blood pressure is higher. Arteries are stiffer due to atherosclerosis, and they are not able to compensate as well for hypotension. Heart muscle and valve issues can affect compensation.
- *Pediatric patients:* Children and young adults have a tremendous ability to compensate for blood loss and may appear relatively normal on a quick scan. A closer look may reveal subtle signs of shock, such as mild tachycardia and tachypnea, pale skin with delayed capillary refilling time, and anxiety. Because of their powerful compensatory mechanisms, children found in decompensated shock represent dire emergencies. Consider typical vital signs by age; compensation can be effective, but decompensation occurs rapidly, so do not hesitate on fluid resuscitation.
- *Pregnancy:* Pregnant patients have an increased blood volume (up to 50%), so they can lose a lot of blood before decompensating and it becomes manifest.
- *Athletes:* Well-trained athletes can have a very low resting heart rate—down to 30 to 40 bpm. A rate of 90 bpm can be a compensatory tachycardia, which can be misinterpreted as a normal value.

CRITICAL THINKING QUESTION

What are some of the platelet inactivators and anticoagulants that are commonly prescribed to patients?

- Platelet inactivators: Aspirin, ticagrelor, prasugrel, and clopidogrel
- Anticoagulants: Warfarin, apixaban, dabigatran, edoxaban, and rivaroxaban

FOR MORE INFORMATION

For more information on the anatomy and physiology of shock, refer to the "Assessment" and "Confounding Factors" sections of Chapter 3: Shock: Pathophysiology of Life and Death in the PHTLS 10th edition main text.

Blood and Blood Products

Blood products offer many advantages. They can restore blood volume, oxygen-carrying capacity, and clotting ability of the blood.

The objectives of blood resuscitation are the restoration of blood volume to restore cellular perfusion but not necessarily restoration of normal blood pressure. The objectives of resuscitation are not the same in every situation (**Figure 4-5**).

- In penetrating trauma with hemorrhage, delaying aggressive fluid resuscitation until definitive control may prevent additional bleeding.

Managing Volume Resuscitation

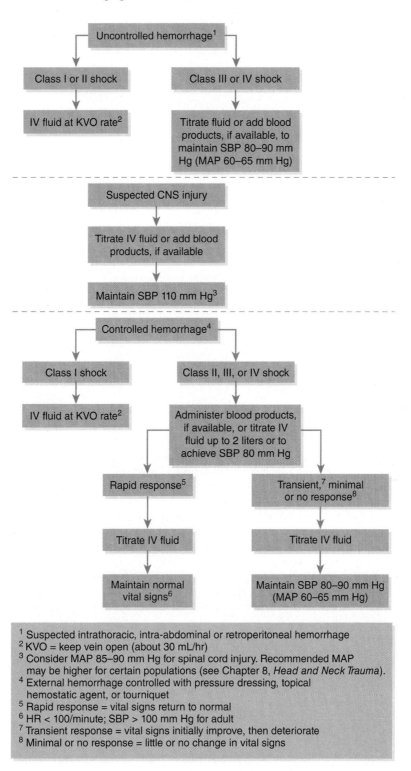

1 Suspected intrathoracic, intra-abdominal or retroperitoneal hemorrhage
2 KVO = keep vein open (about 30 mL/hr)
3 Consider MAP 85–90 mm Hg for spinal cord injury. Recommended MAP
  may be higher for certain populations (see Chapter 8, *Head and Neck Trauma*).
4 External hemorrhage controlled with pressure dressing, topical
  hemostatic agent, or tourniquet
5 Rapid response = vital signs return to normal
6 HR < 100/minute; SBP > 100 mm Hg for adult
7 Transient response = vital signs initially improve, then deteriorate
8 Minimal or no response = little or no change in vital signs

Figure 4-5   A. Algorithm for managing volume resuscitation.

© National Association of Emergency Medical Technicians (NAEMT)

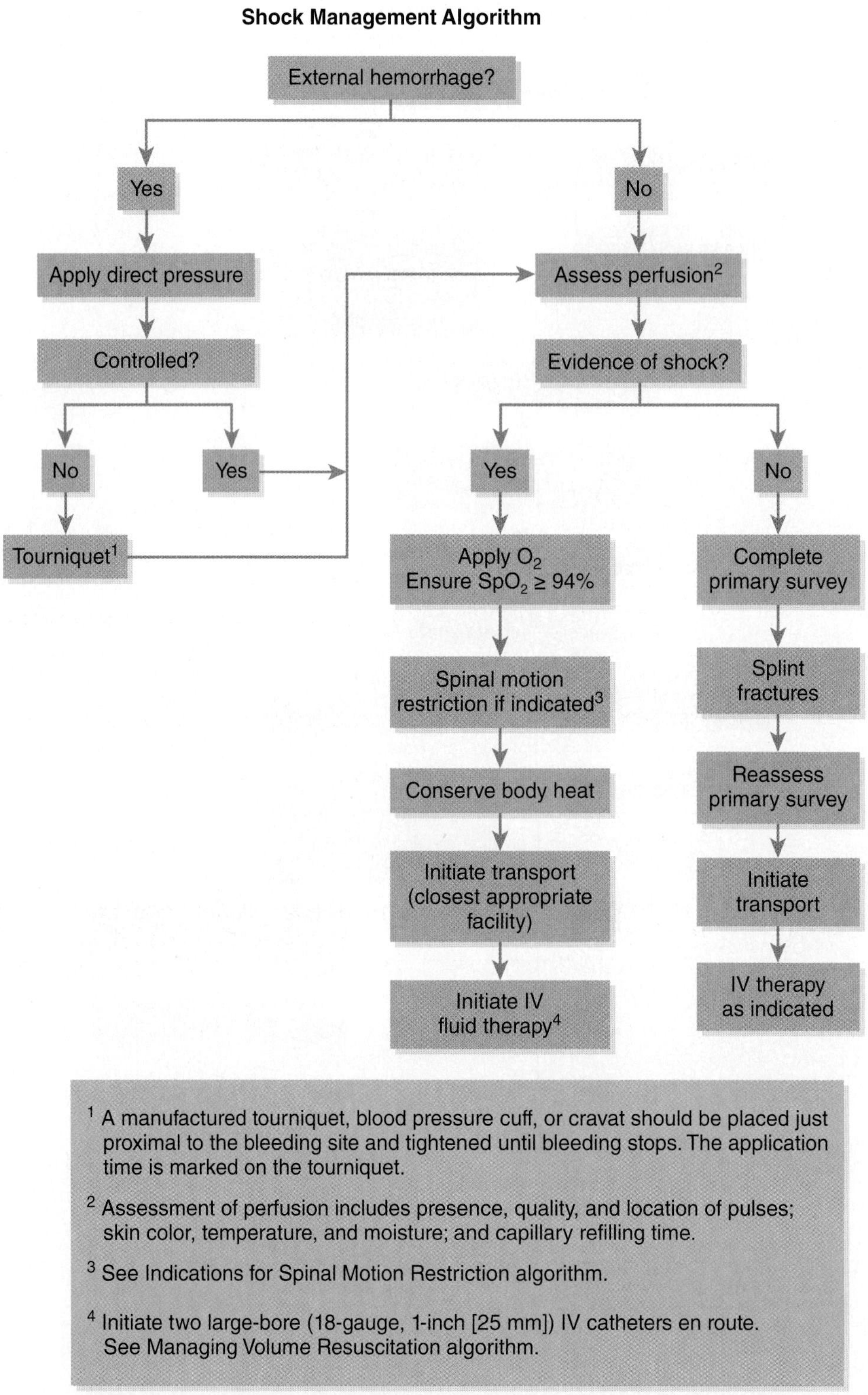

Shock Management Algorithm

External hemorrhage?

Yes → Apply direct pressure → Controlled?

No → Assess perfusion[2] → Evidence of shock?

Controlled? → No → Tourniquet[1]

Controlled? → Yes →

Evidence of shock? → Yes → Apply O₂ Ensure SpO₂ ≥ 94% → Spinal motion restriction if indicated[3] → Conserve body heat → Initiate transport (closest appropriate facility) → Initiate IV fluid therapy[4]

Evidence of shock? → No → Complete primary survey → Splint fractures → Reassess primary survey → Initiate transport → IV therapy as indicated

[1] A manufactured tourniquet, blood pressure cuff, or cravat should be placed just proximal to the bleeding site and tightened until bleeding stops. The application time is marked on the tourniquet.

[2] Assessment of perfusion includes presence, quality, and location of pulses; skin color, temperature, and moisture; and capillary refilling time.

[3] See Indications for Spinal Motion Restriction algorithm.

[4] Initiate two large-bore (18-gauge, 1-inch [25 mm]) IV catheters en route. See Managing Volume Resuscitation algorithm.

Figure 4-5 *(continued)* **B.** Algorithm for managing shock.

© National Association of Emergency Medical Technicians (NAEMT)

- In patients with traumatic brain injury (TBI), a systolic pressure of 110 mm Hg should be achieved to maintain perfusion of the injured brain, even if this means increased bleeding.

Although there is widespread agreement that blood transfusion is more efficient, it presents major logistical issues that are beyond the reach of many EMS systems, although technical advances might change this in the near future.

CRITICAL THINKING QUESTION

How do you tell if altered level of consciousness (LOC) is due to shock or TBI?

■ You cannot always tell at first; however, if the blood pressure is 55/30 mm Hg and oxygen saturation (SpO$_2$) is 70%, altered LOC can be due to hypotension and hypoxemia. If altered LOC persists once hypotension and hypoxemia have been corrected, you must assume TBI is present and set your hemodynamic objectives accordingly.

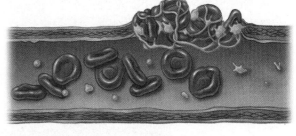

Figure 4-6 Blood clotting involves several enzymes and factors that eventually result in the creation of fibrin molecules, which serve as a matrix to trap platelets and form a plug in a vessel wall to stop bleeding.

© Jones & Bartlett Learning

Blood Products

■ *Whole blood:* Provides endothelial cells for oxygen transport as well as platelets and coagulation factors
■ *RBC concentrates:* Provide volume and RBCs for oxygen transport. Do not contain coagulation factors.
■ *Plasma:* Provides volume and coagulation factors. Lyophilized plasma is the most practical product to handle at present.

More Research Required

Additional research is underway to determine appropriate indications for the use of prehospital TXA, including use in TBI patients, because not all studies have demonstrated a definitive benefit.

Current tactical casualty care guidelines for use in the military and civilian tactical EMS communities endorse a one-time dose of 2 g of TXA given slowly via IV or IO push for:

- Patients who will likely need a blood transfusion (i.e., hemorrhagic shock, elevated lactate, one or more major amputations, penetrating torso trauma, or evidence of severe bleeding)
- Patients with signs of a significant TBI (i.e., altered mental status associated with blast injury or blunt trauma)
- Presentation no later than 3 hours after injury

FOR MORE INFORMATION

Refer to the "Volume Resuscitation" section of Chapter 3: Shock: Pathophysiology of Life and Death in the PHTLS 10th edition main text.

Warning!

■ Rapid IV push of TXA may cause hypotension.
■ If there is a new-onset drop in blood pressure during the infusion, *slow it down!*

Tranexamic Acid

Tranexamic acid (TXA) (an antifibrinolytic agent) is an analog of the amino acid lysine and has been used for many decades to decrease bleeding in certain patient groups. When the coagulation cascade is activated to form a blood clot as a result of an injury, the process of breaking down the blood clot begins at the same time (**Figure 4-6**). Properties of TXA include:

- Interference with the breakdown process to maintain and stabilize newly formed blood clots
- Anti-inflammatory effect

Multiple studies have shown that TXA may improve survival for severely injured trauma patients. TXA appears to be most effective when given early (i.e., < 3 hours after injury) and when patients are severely injured (i.e., hypotensive, tachycardic).

TXA Side Effects

■ Nausea, vomiting, diarrhea
■ Visual disturbances
■ Possible increase in risk of postinjury blood clots
■ Hypotension is possible if given too rapidly as an IV bolus

CASE STUDY: DETAILED ASSESSMENT

Vital Signs:

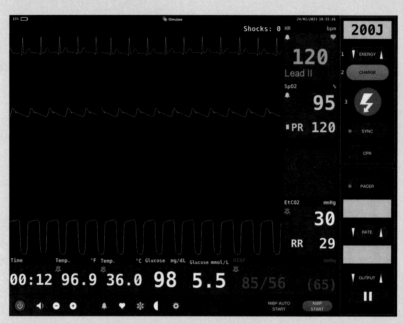

Secondary Assessment:

Detailed Physical Exam

HEENT:

PERRL

Heart and Lungs:

Regular, equal lung sounds

Neuro:

Conscious
GCS 14 (E4, V4, M6)

Abdomen and Pelvis:

Pelvis is tender to palpation. Guarding on palpation of abdomen. Abrasion and bruising noted to LUQ

Upper Extremities:

Bruising and abrasions to arms

Lower Extremities:

No injuries noted

Primary Survey Reassessment:

- **X**—No external hemorrhage; internal bleeding suspected
- **A**—Patent
- **B**—32 breaths/minute, clear equal breath sounds, SpO_2 97%/O_2
- **C**—128 bpm at carotid and radial, skin cool and diaphoretic
- **D**—GCS 14 (E4, V4, M6), moves all extremities
- **E**—Abrasion and bruising noted to LUQ; pelvic tenderness

Questions:

- In this situation, when should the secondary survey, including vital signs, be performed?
- Would the patient's pulse oximetry be reliable at this point?
- Why is the patient breathing rapidly?
- What are the potential life threats at this point?
- What signs of shock are present in this patient?
- Why is it so time sensitive?
- Is loss of red blood cells the only thing that can cause shock?
- Is there a possibility of internal bleeding?

Use Your Tools

Determine the cause of shock through assessment and vital signs:

- Unequal breath sounds when assessing the patient's breathing may indicate a tension pneumothorax.
- Blunt chest trauma with electrocardiogram (ECG) changes may indicate a cardiac contusion.
- High paraplegia or tetraplegia may indicate loss of vascular tone due to a neurologic injury.

QUICK TIP

Trauma patients with a weak radial pulse are 15 times more likely to die than patients with a normal pulse.

FOR MORE INFORMATION

Refer to the "Volume Resuscitation" section of Chapter 3: Shock: Pathophysiology of Life and Death in the PHTLS 10th edition main text.

Blood Loss: External Hemorrhage and Direct Pressure

Why do we check for major bleeding first? Because major bleeding can kill a patient in 3 minutes, and it can usually be controlled by simple direct pressure. Pressing on the bleeding site long enough allows a clot to form and closes the hole in the vessel. This takes about 3 minutes with a hemostatic dressing and up to 10 minutes with normal gauze (provided the patient is not taking any anticoagulant medications). This is why the prehospital algorithm (XABCDE) is different from in-hospital (ABCDE), because patients with major external bleeding will never arrive in the hospital if the problem is not fixed prehospitally.

The ability of the body to respond to and control bleeding depends on:

- The size of the vessel
- The pressure within the vessel
- The presence of clotting factors
- The ability of the injured vessel to go into spasm and reduce the size of the hole and blood flow at the injury site
- The pressure of the surrounding tissue on the vessel at the injury site and any additional pressure provided from the outside

Control of external hemorrhage should proceed in a stepwise fashion, escalating if initial measures fail to control bleeding (**Figure 4-7**).

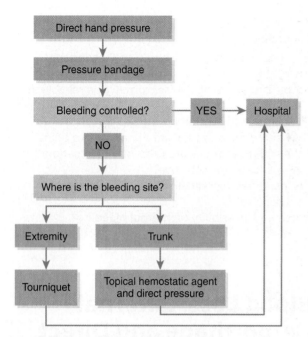

Figure 4-7 Hemorrhage control in the field.
© National Association of Emergency Medical Technicians (NAEMT)

Don't Pop That Clot!

Under normal conditions, a platelet clot can hold a pressure of 80 mm Hg, which is enough for most minor wounds. This has two implications for shock treatment.

1. When you stop the bleeding with direct pressure, pressure should be maintained. Otherwise, if your patient's blood pressure is anything more than 80 mm Hg, the clot will "pop" and bleeding will resume.
2. When you face ongoing (internal) bleeding, if you restore normal blood pressure, you will pop any clot that formed at the bleeding site, increasing bleeding. This is why you should not administer a fluid bolus, because this may "overshoot" the target blood pressure range, resulting in recurrent intrathoracic, intra-abdominal, or retroperitoneal bleeding. Titrate your IV fluids!

Three Critical Reminders

1. When managing a wound with an impaled object, apply pressure on either side of the object rather than over the object. Impaled objects should not be removed in the field because removal of the object could result in uncontrolled internal hemorrhage.

---

2. If hands are required to perform other lifesaving tasks, you can create a pressure (compression) dressing using gauze pads and an elastic roller bandage or a blood pressure cuff inflated until hemorrhage stops. This dressing is placed directly over the bleeding site.
3. Applying direct pressure to exsanguinating hemorrhage takes precedence over insertion of IV lines and fluid resuscitation.

If the dressing becomes soaked with blood, it means that a clot has not formed on the hole in the vessel. Pressure should be maintained because the first clot formed by platelets can only hold a pressure of about 80 mm Hg (the infamous "pop-a-clot" pressure). If the patient's blood pressure is greater than that, the clot will "pop," and bleeding will resume as soon as you let go. Once the bleeding stops, apply a pressure dressing without releasing pressure until the dressing is completely secured.

Volume Resuscitation

There are two general categories of fluid resuscitation products for the management of trauma patients (**Figure 4-8**):

- Blood
  - Packed RBCs (PRBCs)
  - Whole blood
  - Reconstituted whole blood as blood products
  - Plasma
  - Additional blood component therapy
- IV solutions
  - Crystalloid solutions
  - Hypertonic fluid
    - 7% saline
    - 3% saline
  - Colloid solutions (not recommended for prehospital use)
  - Blood substitutes

Because of its ability to transport oxygen and to clot, blood (or blood products) remains the fluid of choice for the resuscitation of a patient in severe hemorrhagic shock.

The rationale for using crystalloids is that because the cardiovascular system is a pump, it needs some volume to work, and crystalloids and colloids can help with that. The downside is dilution of blood components, especially clotting factors, so if you are using crystalloids, only give as much as needed.

The goal of fluid resuscitation is to improve perfusion—restoring a radial pulse and improving mentation.

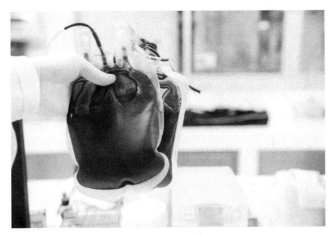

A

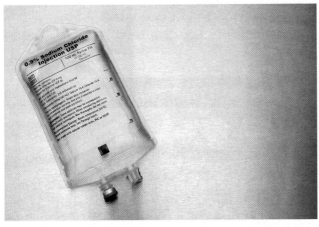

B

Figure 4-8 A. Blood bags. **B.** Saline solution.

A: © Schira/Shutterstock; B: © AlteredR/Shutterstock

Know Your Fluids

- Crystalloid isotonic fluids act as effective volume expanders for a short time, but they do not carry oxygen.
  - NaCl 0.9% (normal saline, or NS)
  - Lactated Ringer solution
    · Same amount of sodium as plasma; provides 1:3 volume expansion (2/3 will exit into the extravascular space)
- Colloids are big molecules that will stay in the intravascular compartment; provides 1:1 volume expansion.
  - Hextend
  - Hetastarch
- Blood products provide 1:1 volume expansion, transport oxygen to the tissues, and prevent coagulopathy.
  - Plasma
  - Whole blood

Titrating Trauma Fluid Resuscitation in the Field

- Avoid "popping the clot."
- Superficial wounds do not require immediate IV access or fluid resuscitation.
- If the patient has appropriate mental status and palpable radial pulse, venous access should be limited to a saline lock.
- If the patient has poor mental status or absent radial pulse, IV access and a 250-mL bolus should be administered.
  - Continue to repeat bolus if no response.
  - Discontinue fluids to a saline lock if a response is noted.
- Patients with head injuries should have fluids titrated to a systolic blood pressure of 110 mm Hg.

Managing Volume in Patients with Signs of Shock and Ongoing Bleeding

Give just enough fluid to maintain perfusion. If systolic BP < 80 mm Hg or absent radial pulse, titrate fluid to have a radial pulse or a systolic blood pressure of 80 to 90 mm Hg (mean arterial pressure [MAP] about 65) and administer TXA when possible. In patients with head trauma, titrate fluids to a systolic blood pressure of at least 110 mm Hg.

QUICK TIP

Remember that a platelet clot can hold up to 80 mm Hg of pressure. If the pressure exceeds this value, all clots already formed inside the body will pop, and bleeding will increase further. A pressure of 80 to 90 mm Hg should maintain adequate perfusion to the kidneys with less risk of worsening internal hemorrhage.

QUICK TIP

Any IV fluid given to a patient in shock should be warm, not room temperature or cold. The ideal temperature for such fluids is 102°F (39°C).

Hypothermia

The combination of coagulopathy, acidosis, and hypothermia is frequently described as the lethal triad. The components are markers of anaerobic metabolism and loss of energy production, and interventions must happen quickly.

Cells work within a finite range of temperature, nominally within a degree of 98.6°F (37°C). If a patient becomes hypothermic, there is increased oxygen demand for the cells to maintain normal temperature (such as shivering).

Hypothermia is a concern because it affects cellular functions and clotting is diminished. In the field, be sure to maintain normothermia, including keeping the patient covered even when exposing to complete an assessment.

CRITICAL THINKING QUESTIONS

What does rapid transport mean?

- It means rapidly assessing and packaging the patient for transport to the appropriate facility (trauma center). The goal is to have an on-scene time of less than 10 minutes.

Should you delay transport to obtain IV access?

- No, delaying transport to start an IV is futile. Obtaining IV access can be done during transport; an 18-gauge or larger IV is desirable for blood administration.

What are the components of basic shock treatment?

- Bleeding control, oxygenation, and maintaining normothermia are all important.

CASE STUDY: TRANSPORT AND ONGOING MANAGEMENT

The patient is packaged and is ready for transport. An IV is established. During transport, the patient's body heat is maintained with a blanket and warm environment. Vitals are reassessed throughout transport.

Questions:

- Does this patient require spinal stabilization?
- What is your transport destination?
- What interventions will you perform en route?

CASE STUDY: WRAP-UP

The patient was transported to a Level I trauma center with surgical capability. Once in the trauma center, the patient was found to have a pelvic ring fracture and ruptured spleen with internal bleeding. He underwent a surgical splenectomy and recovered completely.

Question:

- What are the future implications for the patient after having a splenectomy?

SUMMARY

- Stop the bleeding! No IV fluid is better than the patient's blood.

- Shock = inadequate cellular perfusion.

- Optimize oxygenation.

- Evaluate the need for volume replacement and consider available options.

- Maintain normothermia.

- Rapid transport for patients with suspected internal bleeding is paramount.

CASE STUDY RECAP

Dispatch

What potential injuries do you expect this patient to have based on the available information?

- Head trauma, internal and/or external hemorrhage, thoracic trauma, spinal cord injury, shock, fractures to extremities, abrasions

Initial Impression	
What are the scene safety concerns?	■ Traffic hazards, road visibility (twisting, rural road), fuel leaks

Primary Survey	
What are the potential life threats given the mechanism of injury and primary survey results?	■ Possible internal injury, shock
Why is it important to check airway and breathing in this patient?	■ If there is no airway and breathing, then oxygen is not being carried by the blood. ■ Given the mechanism of injury, it is important to rule out other injuries, such as tension pneumothorax.
Which organ(s) in the LUQ could cause severe internal bleeding?	■ The spleen is highly vascular and can result in severe bleeding if it is ruptured.

Detailed Assessment	
In this situation, when should the secondary survey, including vital signs, be performed?	■ Secondary survey may be delayed due to the presence of life threats and associated treatment. ■ If other EMS personnel are present, secondary and vitals may be performed simultaneously with management of the life threats.
Would the patient's pulse oximetry be reliable at this point?	■ Pulse oximetry relies on pulsatile flow of blood in the capillaries, so diminished blood flow and loss of RBCs render pulse oximetry unreliable. ■ Look at the patient, and do not depend on machines that may not provide an accurate clinical picture due to decreased blood pressure and decreased peripheral circulation.
Why is the patient breathing rapidly?	■ It could be a result of the stress of the situation, and it could also be due to shock from blood loss (rapid breathing compensating for lactic acid production).
What are the potential life threats at this point?	■ The abrasion and hematoma to the LUQ may indicate internal bleeding. ■ Pelvic tenderness likely indicates pelvic ring fracture, which may be accompanied by internal bleeding.
What signs of shock are present in this patient?	■ Rapid breathing, rapid heart rate, altered mental status, cool skin, low BP
Why is it so time sensitive?	■ The lack of oxygen supply to the cells leads to anaerobic metabolism within a few minutes.
Is loss of RBCs the only thing that can cause shock?	■ No, any mechanism that impedes oxygen delivery to the cells can cause shock, such as tension pneumothorax or cardiac tamponade.
Is there a possibility of internal bleeding?	■ There is a high probability given the mechanism of injury, the abrasion and bruising to the LUQ, pelvic tenderness, and the signs of shock.

Transport and Ongoing Management	
Does this patient require spinal stabilization?	▪ Yes, given the mechanism of injury and decreasing LOC.
What is your transport destination?	▪ A Level I trauma center with surgical capability, because internal hemorrhage and shock are suspected.
What interventions will you perform en route?	▪ You apply a pelvic binder, establish spinal motion restriction, transfer the patient to the ambulance, and begin transport to the closest trauma center. ▪ En route, you apply oxygen at 2 L/minute via nonrebreather mask with ETCO₂ monitoring. ▪ You place two 18-gauge IV lines, giving only enough fluid to maintain a systolic BP of > 90 mm Hg. ▪ Due to the patient's hemodynamics and the potential for internal hemorrhage, you note the patient is a candidate for TXA administration. ▪ During transport, the patient's body heat is maintained with a blanket and warm environment. ▪ Vitals are reassessed throughout transport.
Wrap-Up	
What are the future implications for the patient after having a splenectomy?	▪ The spleen is an important component of the immune system; thus, the patient will be at an increased risk for infection.

STUDY QUESTIONS

1. Your partner is compressing the bleeding site of a male patient who was stabbed multiple times in the left chest. The bleeding seems to be controlled, yet the patient becomes combative. He is pale and is breathing rapidly, yet states that he "can't breathe" and feels that he is about to die. Your next step in patient management is to:
   A. start assisted ventilation.
   B. give high-flow oxygen.
   C. decompress the left chest.
   D. give a 250-mL fluid bolus.

2. The patient's respiration improves markedly, but he remains confused. He has an absent radial pulse, and his carotid pulse is fast and thready. Your partner asks if he can let the compression go to put in an IV. How should you respond?
   A. "Oh yes, that's a great idea!"
   B. "Yes, but we have to immobilize him first."
   C. "Take a blood pressure first to see if he needs an IV."
   D. "No, keep the pressure and let's get out of here!"

3. While en route to the hospital, you manage to put an 18-gauge IV in the right arm. Your patient is still confused, and you still have no radial pulse. Your next move is to:
   A. give 1-L fluid bolus.
   B. give one 250-mL fluid bolus, and then stop.
   C. give fluid until you get a radial pulse.
   D. administer TXA.

4. After 400 mL of lactated Ringer solution, you get a radial pulse and his level of consciousness improves. The monitor shows heart rate 110 beats/minute, blood pressure 85/60 mm Hg, SpO₂ 95%, ventilation rate 25 breaths/minute. What should you do?
   A. Give an additional 500 mL of lactated Ringer solution.
   B. Stop fluids and give 2 g of TXA.
   C. Give TXA and 500 mL of normal saline.
   D. Give 2 mg of morphine for analgesia.

5. You now perform a secondary survey. You notice a sternotomy scar. Your patient tells you he is on oral clopidogrel since he had a coronary artery bypass graft 2 years ago. Is this information useful?
    A. No, he should stop talking and breathe.
    B. Yes, he should see a cardiologist once in the local hospital.
    C. Yes, he will need platelets and a heart surgeon ASAP.
    D. Yes, you should raise his blood pressure up to 130 mm Hg systolic.

ANSWER KEY

Question 1: C
After X come A and B. You can quickly auscultate the lungs (pneumothorax is almost certain with multiple stabs in the chest) and decompress the chest. Decompressing a tension pneumothorax is the quickest way to treat shock.

Question 2: D
This patient is likely in decompensated shock with internal bleeding, so rapid transport is the next priority. You should maintain pressure on the wound, because having massive external bleeding start up again is the last thing you want in this situation.

Question 3: C
Now is the time to titrate IV fluids to restore tissue perfusion. Giving 1 liter blindly could overshoot your target pressure and reinforce internal bleeding. TXA is not a priority, although it can run parallel to fluids.

Question 4: B
The patient does not need more fluids right now. Giving morphine in a shocked patient is a risky move and could lead to dangerous hypotension.

Question 5: C
Because he is on clopidogrel, his platelets are out of order for at least 5 days, so he will require urgent platelet transfusion.

REFERENCES AND FURTHER READING

National Association of Emergency Medical Technicians. *PHTLS: Prehospital Trauma Life Support.* 10th ed. Burlington, MA: Public Safety Group; 2023.

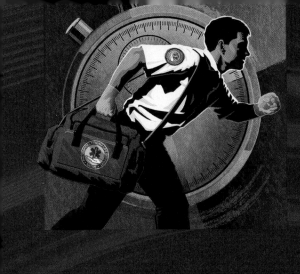

D—Disability: Traumatic Brain Injury (TBI)

LESSON OBJECTIVES

- Explain the pathophysiology, signs, and symptoms of traumatic brain injury (TBI).
- Discuss the difference between primary and secondary TBI.
- Identify mechanisms of injury with a high index of suspicion for TBI.
- Demonstrate the assessment and management of a patient with a TBI.
- Identify special considerations in geriatric and pediatric patients with TBI.

Introduction

Traumatic brain injury (TBI) is a worldwide public health problem that affects over 10 million people annually across the globe. In the United States, TBI is a leading cause of injury-related death and disability, and it is the most frequent cause of death and disability among children worldwide, with more than 3 million children sustaining brain injuries yearly. In 2019 there were over 223,135 TBI-related hospitalizations; in 2020 there were 64,362 TBI-related deaths. This does not include the TBIs that are treated in the emergency department and then discharged, those treated in primary care or urgent care settings, and those that go untreated. That's more than 611 TBI-related admissions and 176 TBI-related deaths per day.

Patients with TBI can be some of the most challenging trauma patients to treat. They may be combative, and attempts to manage the airway can be difficult because of clenched jaw muscles and vomiting. Assessment can be further hindered by shock from other injuries or drug and/or alcohol intoxication. Occasionally, serious intracranial injuries are present but there is minimal or no external evidence of trauma.

Skilled care in the prehospital setting focuses on ensuring the adequate delivery of oxygen and nutrients to the brain and rapidly identifying patients at risk for herniation and elevated intracranial pressure. This approach decreases mortality and reduces the incidence of permanent neurologic disability. Our goal when treating TBI is to keep further harm from occurring to even a single brain cell and to establish conditions optimal for healing and recovery.

Basic Anatomy

Three things exist within the cranial cavity: blood, cerebrospinal fluid (CSF), and brain matter (**Figure 5A-1**). All three of these components exist within their own capsule:

1. Brain within the skull
2. Blood within the capillaries
3. Cerebrospinal fluid within the ventricles, subarachnoid space, and spinal cord

There is only room for a specific amount of each within the rigid cranial vault. The Monro-Kellie doctrine states that the sum of the volume of brain tissue, blood, and CSF must remain constant in patients with an intact skull. Therefore, an increase in one component (such as from a hematoma, cerebral swelling, or tumor) must cause a decrease in one or two of the other components or the intracranial pressure (ICP) will increase.

> ### FOR MORE INFORMATION
>
> *Refer to the "Anatomy" section of Chapter 8: Head and Neck Trauma in the PHTLS 10th edition main text.*

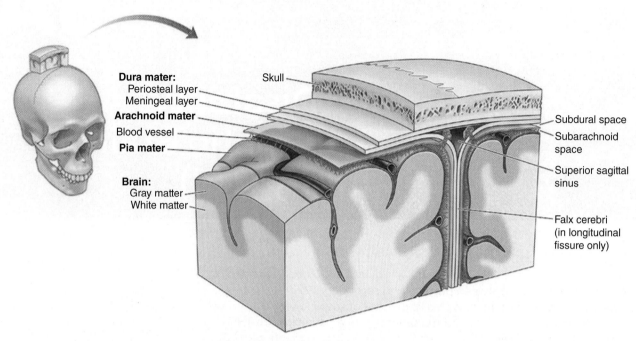

Figure 5A-1 Basic anatomy of the brain, including meningeal coverings.
Courtesy of the American College of Surgeons.

CASE STUDY: DISPATCH

You and your partner are dispatched to a motor vehicle collision with a power pole. It is a clear, hot, summer day with a temperature of 87°F (30.5°C).

One vehicle is involved, with one older adult patient in the driver's seat, and significant damage to the front of the vehicle. Witnesses state the patient veered off the road and struck the pole head-on without slowing down. Speed limit is 45 mph (72.4 kph) for this section of road. The airbag did not deploy, and the patient appears to be wearing a shoulder and lap belt.

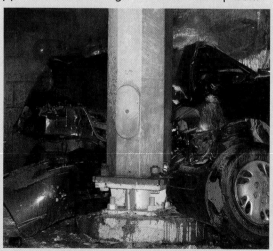

© Jack Dagley Photography/Shutterstock

The fire department is already on scene and advises you the scene is safe. You are currently 20 minutes from a Level I trauma center and 5 minutes from a free-standing emergency department.

Questions:
- Is the scene safe?
- How and where should you park your ambulance?
- Is the power pole stable, and/or is there a threat of electrocution from power lines?
- Should the local power company be present?
- How does the knowledge that the airbag has not deployed affect your approach?
- What are the potential injuries to the patient?

Physiology

Oxygen and Cerebral Blood Flow

The brain has high oxygen requirements. Decreased levels of oxygen (hypoxia) cause major vasodilation in an effort to increase cerebral blood flow. This response typically doesn't occur until the arterial oxygen partial pressure (PaO_2) falls below 50 mm Hg, but when it does, it can further increase brain volume and therefore intracranial pressure.

Pulse oximetry is an important tool for monitoring the oxygen status of a patient with a TBI because it measures the amount of red blood cells bound by oxygen. The prehospital practitioner should make every effort to minimize blood loss to ensure sufficient red blood cells to meet the body's metabolic needs.

The 4- to 6-Minute Window

Brief periods of hypo-oxygenation can be very harmful to the patient with a brain injury. Irreversible brain damage can occur after only 4 to 6 minutes of arterial desaturation in the injured brain.

Hyperoxia has also been shown to be harmful when it happens for long periods of time; however, hypoxia has been shown to be the more damaging of the two. A pulse oximetry reading of > 94% should be maintained. The minimal goal is 90%. Remember that O_2 saturation is not always reliable but is indicated for monitoring oxygenation on all trauma patients.

Carbon Dioxide and Cerebral Blood Flow

The cerebral blood vessels respond to changes in arterial carbon dioxide levels by either constricting or dilating. Decreased levels of carbon dioxide (hypocapnia) result in vasoconstriction, whereas elevated levels (hypercapnia) cause vasodilation.

Hyperventilation reduces the $PaCO_2$ by increasing the rate at which carbon dioxide gets blown off by the lungs. The resulting hypocapnia changes the acid–base balance in the brain, resulting in vasoconstriction. This reduces the intravascular volume of the brain, reducing cerebral blood volume and, therefore, often ICP. However, this comes at a price, which is reduced cerebral perfusion.

Ventilation

Ventilation is the act of air and oxygen entering and exiting the body. When we say we assist ventilations on a patient, we use a device to circulate air in and out. The addition of oxygen supports oxygenation measured by pulse oximetry.

The ventilatory rate of a patient with a TBI should be maintained between 10 and 20 breaths per minute. Waveform capnography is a valuable tool in assessing a patient's ventilatory status. It should be maintained between 35 and 40 mm Hg. The lower the value in CO_2, the smaller the blood vessels get, thus impeding blood flow to the brain and starving the brain of oxygen. The higher the value in CO_2, the larger the blood vessels get, increasing blood flow to the brain and by default increasing ICP.

While monitoring waveform capnography, the ventilatory rate should be adjusted to keep the end-tidal carbon dioxide ($ETCO_2$) ideally within 35 to 40 mm Hg, but no less than 30 mm Hg. Remember to maximize the volume and control CO_2 with the ventilatory rate. Note the suggested ventilatory rate for different age groups:

- *Adult:* 20 breaths/minute
- *Child:* 25 breaths/minute
- *Infant:* (< 1 yr) 30 breaths/minute

CRITICAL THINKING QUESTIONS

Why is airway management important in a patient with TBI?

- Hypoxia is a major concern with a TBI. Irreversible brain damage can occur after only 4 to 6 minutes of arterial desaturation in the injured brain. A significant number of patients with TBI present with low or inadequate oxygen saturation (SpO_2), which may be missed without the use of pulse oximetry.
- You must ensure adequate circulation by minimizing blood loss and ensure adequate oxygenation by maintaining a patent airway and adequate ventilation.

Does SpO_2 or $ETCO_2$ tell us more about the ventilatory status of a patient with TBI?

- Remember that a ventilatory rate between 10 and 20 breaths/minute in an adult patient with TBI and an oxygen saturation rate of 94% or greater are the most important indicators of ventilation and perfusion. $ETCO_2$ isn't always reliable in an unstable patient and provides only a rough estimate of hypoventilation or hyperventilation. Nonetheless, you should try to maintain an $ETCO_2$ between 35 and 40 mm Hg for a patient with TBI.

FOR MORE INFORMATION

Refer to the "Physiology" and "Pathophysiology" sections of Chapter 8: Head and Neck Trauma in the PHTLS 10th edition main text.

CASE STUDY: INITIAL IMPRESSION

Fire department is on scene and has determined that the scene is safe. The airbag has been disarmed, there is no threat from the power pole, and traffic is adequately controlled.

There appears to be only one patient, an older adult male (age > 65) who is awake and sitting in the driver's seat. His seat belt is still in place, he is clutching his chest, and he has a large hematoma to the forehead and complaint of headache. There is significant damage to the front of the vehicle. There is a high index of suspicion for some type of head injury.

Questions:
- Based on what you know, what kinds of forces were exerted on the driver of the vehicle?
- What three impacts were involved?

Primary Versus Secondary Brain Injury

TBI can be divided into two categories: primary and secondary.

Primary Brain Injury

Primary brain injury occurs at the time of the original insult and is any injury that occurs due to the initial trauma. This includes injury to the brain, its coverings, and associated vascular structures.

Primary brain injuries include:

- Brain contusions
- Hemorrhages
- Damage to nerves and brain vessels

Because neural tissue doesn't regenerate well and it can't really be repaired, there won't be much recovery of the structure and function lost due to primary injury.

Secondary Brain Injury

Injured brain tissue is extremely susceptible to further injury, and many secondary injuries can lead to the death of brain cells that would have otherwise survived. Secondary brain injury is continued injury to structures that occurs after the initial impact. Once an injury occurs, a number of processes kick in, making the brain vulnerable to further injury for hours to even weeks after the initial insult. *The main goal in the prehospital management of TBI is to identify and limit or stop these secondary injury mechanisms.*

The Hidden Villain

The secondary effects of traumatic brain injury are insidious and there's often significant, ongoing damage that isn't immediately apparent. These effects play a major role in death and disability after TBIs. By understanding what type of secondary injury is likely to occur as a result of the primary trauma, we can prepare for and intervene to correct these complications or prevent them from occurring.

Two other important causes of secondary injury are *hypoxia* and *hypotension*. Unrecognized and untreated hypoxia and hypotension are as harmful to the injured brain as elevated ICP. In addition, impaired oxygen or glucose delivery to an injured brain is more devastating than in the normal brain. Therefore, avoiding and/or treating hypoxia and hypotension as much as possible is critical.

Hypotension

Many patients with TBI sustain other injuries, often involving hemorrhage and subsequent hypotension. Fluid resuscitation, as well as rapid definitive treatment of these injuries to prevent hypotension, is important in mitigating the risk of secondary injury. Higher cerebral perfusion pressures are required to maintain adequate cerebral blood flow.

Severely injured areas of the brain can lose almost all ability to autoregulate as the blood vessels become dilated, causing hyperemia and shunting of blood toward the most severely injured brain areas and away from areas that could still be saved by adequate perfusion. Aggressive hyperventilation can further threaten cerebral blood flow and compound the ischemic threat by constricting blood vessels to both compromised and unaffected areas of the brain.

QUICK TIP

Too much oxygen, or hyperoxia, is associated with worse outcomes. One hundred percent oxygen can cause cerebral vasoconstriction, which can alter brain metabolism.

This combination of physiologic downregulation, shunting, and hemorrhagic shock creates multiple ischemic threats to the salvageable areas of the brain and makes the aggressive management of hypotension an essential part of the management of TBI. For this reason, an aggressive approach in the prehospital environment, with prehospital fluid resuscitation aimed at keeping the systolic blood pressure above 110 mm Hg, is essential to limiting secondary injury in a brain-injured patient.

In the national TBI database, the two most significant predictors of poor outcome from TBI were:

- The amount of time spent with an ICP greater than 20 mm Hg.
- The amount of time spent with a systolic blood pressure less than 90 mm Hg.

Several studies have confirmed the profound impact of low systolic blood pressure on the outcome after TBI.

CASE STUDY: PRIMARY SURVEY

- **X**—No obvious external life-threatening hemorrhage.
- **A**—Patent without obstruction; patient is speaking without difficulty.
- **B**—RR 20 breaths/minute with clear bilateral breath sounds, SpO$_2$ 94%.
- **C**—Skin is warm and flushed; pulse is strong and present radially at 75 bpm.
- **D**—Awake but slightly confused. Patient cannot remember events leading to collision. GCS 13 (E3, V4, M6); pupils are 3 mm round and reactive.
- **E**—You expose to find sternal redness and a palpable implant to left upper chest.

Questions:

- Is there a need for hemorrhage control?
- Is airway management needed?
- Is spinal motion restriction indicated?
- Is the patient a reliable source for clearing the cervical spine?
- What special considerations may be present for this patient?
- Could this patient have a traumatic brain injury?

FOR MORE INFORMATION

Refer to the "Pathophysiology of Traumatic Brain Injury: Secondary Brain Injury" section of Chapter 8: Head and Neck Trauma in the PHTLS 10th edition main text.

Seizures

A patient with acute TBI is at risk for seizures for several reasons:

- Hypoxia from airway or breathing problems can cause generalized seizure activity, as can hypoglycemia and electrolyte abnormalities.
- Ischemic or damaged brain tissue can produce grand mal seizures or status epilepticus.
- Seizures can aggravate preexisting hypoxia.
- Seizures can further harm the injured brain because the neuronal activity associated with generalized seizures rapidly depletes oxygen and glucose levels, which further worsens cerebral ischemia.

Types of Traumatic Brain Injury

Mild TBIs/Concussions

Mild TBIs, including *concussions*, are the most common type of traumatic brain injury. They are caused by a strong force striking the head (**Figure 5A-2**). Symptoms can range from mild to severe. Symptoms lasting over a month are considered *postconcussion syndrome*. Severe headache, dizziness, nausea, and vomiting frequently accompany a concussion. Patients exhibiting signs of concussion, especially patients with nausea, vomiting, or neurologic findings on secondary survey, should be immediately transported for further evaluation.

The formal diagnosis of a concussion will be made in the hospital once the patient has been evaluated and a head CT scan result shows no observable intracranial pathology. Concussion requires a thorough follow-up, because the symptoms and the susceptibility to secondary injury can last for weeks.

"Complicated mild TBI," characterized by microhemorrhage and contusion, may present with postconcussive symptoms (**Table 5A-1**) lasting longer than the traditional recovery period of 2 to 4 weeks.

Contusions

Contusions are bruises on the brain and are often seen with a concussion. They are a mild form of bleeding. Symptoms depend on size and location. Damage to the brain itself may produce cerebral contusions. If the damage includes injury to the blood vessels in the brain, there will be bleeding within the brain, known as intracerebral hematomas (see the following section). Cerebral contusions are common both in patients with

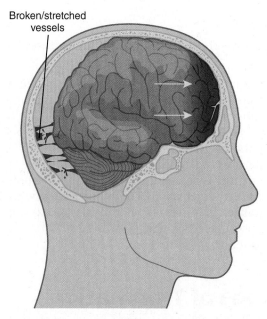

Broken/stretched vessels

Figure 5A-2 As the skull stops its forward motion, the brain continues to move forward. The part of the brain nearest the impact is compressed, bruised, and perhaps even lacerated. The portion farthest from the impact is separated from the skull, with tearing and lacerations of the vessels involved.

© National Association of Emergency Medical Technicians (NAEMT)

Table 5A-1 Common Postconcussive Symptoms	
Categories	**Symptoms**
Vestibular	Imbalance, nausea, dizziness
Sensory	Blurry vision, migraines, tinnitus, photo/phonophobia
Cognitive	Difficulty focusing, forgetfulness
Emotional	Fatigue, insomnia, irritability, depression

Data from Quinn DK, Mayer AR, Master CL, Fann JR. Prolonged postconcussive symptoms. *Am J Psychiatry.* 2018;175(2):103-111. doi:10.1176/appi.ajp.2017.17020235

severe brain injuries and in those with moderate head injuries. Contusions often occur in locations far from the site of impact, often on the opposite side of the brain (coup-contrecoup injury—see "Coup-Contrecoup Brain Injury" later in this chapter).

Cerebral contusions often take 12 to 24 hours to appear on CT scans. The only clue to their presence may be a depressed Glasgow Coma Scale (GCS) score. These contusions can increase dramatically in patients taking anticoagulants or antiplatelets.

QUICK TIP

Cerebral contusions may cause moderate head injuries to deteriorate to severe head injuries in about 10% of patients.

Intracranial Hemorrhages

Intracranial hemorrhages are bleeding on the surface of the brain or within the brain tissue itself. Hemorrhage occurring in the space surrounding the brain (under the arachnoid membrane) is known as *subarachnoid hemorrhage (SAH)*. Hemorrhage in the cerebral matter is called *intracerebral hemorrhage*. These hemorrhages can be life threatening, but tend to be less severe than other types of TBI.

Blood in the subarachnoid space can't enter the subdural space. Many of the brain's blood vessels are located in the subarachnoid space, so injury to these vessels causes subarachnoid bleeding, a layering of blood beneath the arachnoid membrane on the surface of the brain. This is typically thin and rarely causes mass effect.

SAH usually results from a spontaneous rupture of cerebral aneurysms and causes the sudden onset of the worst headache of the patient's life. Patients usually complain of headaches, which may be severe, as well as nausea, vomiting, and dizziness. In addition, the presence of blood in the subarachnoid space can cause meningeal signs like pain and stiffness of the neck, visual complaints, and photophobia (aversion to bright light).

Follow My Finger

Bleeding from the posterior communicating artery can cause oculomotor nerve abnormalities or loss of movement on the ipsilateral (same) side; the affected eye will look down and outward, and patients can't lift their eyelids. These patients may also develop seizures, although seizure development is more common in cerebral aneurysm rupture or arteriovenous malformations.

Intracranial Hematomas

Intracranial hematomas are collections of blood outside the blood vessels within the skull. *Epidural hematomas* are bleeding between the inside of the skull and the outer covering of the brain (dura). *Subdural hematomas* are bleeding between the brain and its outermost lining (dura). *Intracerebral hematoma*, or intraparenchymal hemorrhage, is bleeding that occurs in the functional tissue of the brain consisting of neurons and glial cells. Hematomas may take days to develop after a head injury, requiring a high index of suspicion by the prehospital practitioner.

Because the signs and symptoms of each hematoma have definite overlap, specific diagnosis in the prehospital setting (as well as the ED) is almost impossible. You may suspect a particular type of hematoma based on the characteristic clinical presentation, but a definitive diagnosis can be made only after a CT scan. Because these hematomas occupy space inside the rigid skull, they may produce rapid increases in ICP, especially if they're sizable.

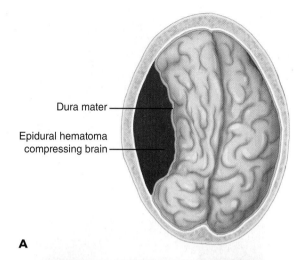

A

Older Noggin, Greater Risk

In a geriatric patient:

- Veins are more susceptible to tearing, increasing the risk of a subdural hematoma from minor blunt trauma.
- Brain atrophy results in increased space in the cranial vault.
- A larger volume of blood may accumulate before outward signs of increased intracranial pressure are present.

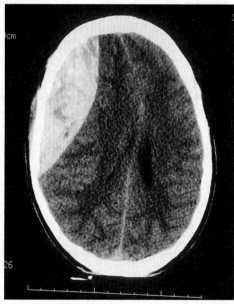

B

Figure 5A-3 A. Epidural hematoma. **B.** CT scan of epidural hematoma.

A. © National Association of Emergency Medical Technicians (NAEMT); **B.** Courtesy of Peter T. Pons, MD, FACEP.

Epidural Hematoma

Epidural hematomas often result from a low-velocity blow to the temporal bone, such as the impact from a punch or baseball. A fracture of this thin bone damages the middle meningeal artery, which results in arterial bleeding that collects between the skull and dura mater. This high-pressure arterial blood can start to dissect, or peel, the dura off of the inner table of the skull, creating an epidural space full of blood. The principal threat to the brain is from the expanding mass of blood displacing the brain and threatening herniation (**Figure 5A-3**).

The classic sign for an epidural hematoma is a patient experiencing a brief loss of consciousness, then regaining consciousness, and then experiencing a rapid decline in consciousness. During the period of consciousness (the lucid interval) the patient may be oriented, lethargic, or confused and may complain of a headache. A patient who experiences a lucid interval,

followed by a decline in GCS score, needs emergency evaluation. As a patient's consciousness worsens, the physical examination may reveal a dilated and sluggish or nonreactive pupil, most commonly on the ipsilateral (same) side of the herniation.

Subdural Hematoma

In addition to being more common than epidural hematomas, subdural hematomas differ in etiology, location, and prognosis. Unlike the epidural hematoma, which is caused by arterial hemorrhage, a subdural hematoma generally results from a venous bleed and is associated with direct brain injury. In this case, bridging veins are torn during a violent blow to the head. Blood collects

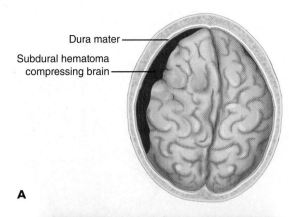

Dura mater

Subdural hematoma compressing brain

A

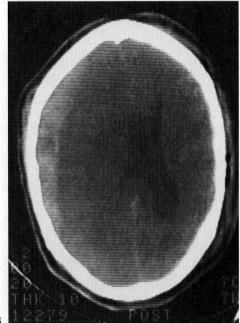

B

Figure 5A-4 **A.** Subdural hematoma. **B.** CT scan of subdural hematoma.

A. © National Association of Emergency Medical Technicians (NAEMT); **B.** Courtesy of Peter T. Pons, MD, FACEP.

in the subdural space, between the dura mater and the underlying arachnoid membrane (**Figure 5A-4**).

Subdural hematomas present in two different ways:

1. In patients who've experienced significant trauma, the tearing of the bridging veins results in a rapid accumulation of blood in the subdural space, with rapid onset of mass effect. These patients will exhibit an acutely depressed mental status and will need immediate transport to an appropriate receiving facility for CT scan, ICP monitoring and management, and possibly surgery.

2. Clinically occult subdural hematomas can also occur. In older adults or patients with chronic diseases, the subdural space enlarges due to brain atrophy. Blood may accumulate in the subdural space without causing mass effect

and can remain asymptomatic for a long time. Such subdural hematomas can occur during falls in older adults or during minor trauma.

Because the onset of the mass effect is gradual, the patient doesn't have the dramatic signs associated with an acute subdural hematoma. Instead, the patient is more likely to present with headache, visual disturbances, personality changes, difficulty speaking (dysarthria), and hemiparesis or hemiplegia that is slow to progress. A chronic subdural hematoma might only be discovered when some of these symptoms become obvious enough to prompt the patient or caregiver to seek help.

> **QUICK TIP**
>
> Prehospital care practitioners frequently encounter these patients when called to facilities that care for chronically ill populations. Because the symptoms are nonspecific, diagnosing a chronic subdural hematoma in the field is rarely possible, and the symptoms may be confused with those of a stroke, infection, dementia, or even a generalized decline in the patient.

Coup-Contrecoup Brain Injury

Coup-contrecoup brain injury is French for "blow" and "counterblow." The coup injury occurs directly at the point of impact. The contrecoup injury occurs on the opposite side of the brain from impact. By this definition, it can be considered two separate injuries. When the skull hits an object or is struck by an object, the brain moves forward and collides with the skull, causing injury. The brain then rebounds and collides with the opposite side of the skull, causing further injury.

Penetrating Brain Injury

A *penetrating brain injury* is most commonly caused by a bullet penetrating the skull, but can be caused by any foreign body. This results in direct trauma to the brain and surrounding structures. Closed, depressed skull fractures may require neurosurgical intervention because the decrease in intracranial space by the encroaching fracture results in increased ICP, and an underlying cerebral injury is often present (**Figure 5A-5**).

Open skull fractures can happen during a particularly forceful impact or a gunshot wound and serve as an entry site for bacteria, predisposing the patient to meningitis. If the dura mater is torn, brain tissue or CSF may leak from an open skull fracture. Because of the risk of meningitis, these wounds require immediate neurosurgical evaluation.

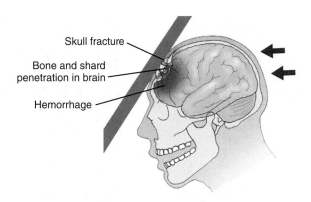

Figure 5A-5 As the skull impacts an object, pieces of bone may be fractured and pushed into the brain.

© National Association of Emergency Medical Technicians (NAEMT)

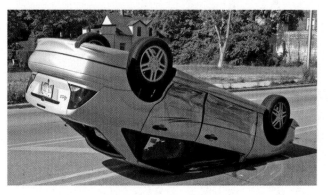

Figure 5A-6 During a rollover, the unrestrained occupant can be wholly or partially ejected from the vehicle or can bounce around inside the vehicle. This action produces multiple and somewhat unpredictable injuries that are often severe.

© Rechitan Sorin/Shutterstock

- Presence of alcohol or unknown substance
- Hypoglycemia
- Dementia

Types of TBI

- Mild TBIs, including concussions
- Contusions (bruise)
- Intracranial hemorrhages
- Intracranial hematomas
- Coup-contrecoup brain injury
- Penetrating brain injury

Mechanisms with High Index of Suspicion

There are three different forces that can cause a traumatic brain injury.

1. Blunt
   - Falls
   - Motor vehicle crash (MVC)
   - Sport-related accident
   - Assault
2. Penetrating
   - Gunshot wound
   - Stabbing
   - Explosive causing projectiles—causes disruption and primary injury to the skull and surrounding tissues
3. Deceleration or shearing force
   - MVC (**Figure 5A-6**)
   - Recreational vehicle collisions

Hypoxia from drowning, hanging, or any asphyxiation can also cause traumatic brain injury due to swelling. Any abnormal finding in Glasgow Coma Scale score or neurologic assessment should alert the prehospital practitioner to the potential for traumatic brain injury.

The prehospital practitioner should not rule out traumatic brain injury in the presence of other masking findings when there is a suspicious mechanism. Examples of masking findings include:

Symptoms of TBI

Not all TBIs present the same or share each listed symptom; the following list should not be considered all-inclusive:

- Cognitive
  - Amnesia
  - Confusion
  - Inability to speak or understand language
- Behavioral
  - Aggression
  - Repetition of words or actions
- Mood
  - Angry
  - Anxious
- Body
  - Dizziness
  - Fainting
- Eyes
  - Dilated pupils (**Figure 5A-7A**)
  - Unequal pupils (**Figure 5A-7B**)
  - Periorbital ecchymosis (referred to as "raccoon eyes" in North America)
  - Blurred vision
- Gastrointestinal
  - Nausea
  - Vomiting
- Other physical findings may include:
  - Persistent headache
  - Temporary moment of clarity
  - Loss of smell
  - Seizures
  - Ringing in ears

Crashes and Falls

Motor vehicle crashes are the leading cause of TBI in patients between 5 and 75 years of age, whereas falls are the leading cause of TBI in pediatric patients up to 4 years of age and in the older adult population.

FOR MORE INFORMATION

Refer to the "Pathophysiology of Traumatic Brain Injury: Primary Brain Injury" section of Chapter 8: Head and Neck Trauma in the PHTLS 10th edition main text.

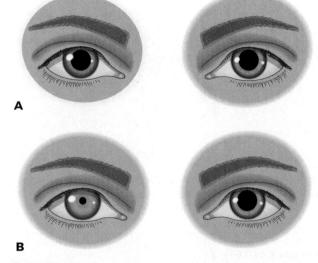

A

B

Figure 5A-7 Dilated (**A**) or unequal pupils (**B**) can be a symptom of TBI.

© Jones & Bartlett Learning

CASE STUDY: DETAILED ASSESSMENT

Primary Survey Reassessment:

- **X**—None.
- **A**—Patent without obstruction, patient is speaking inappropriate words.
- **B**—Patient is breathing 20 times a minute with bilateral breath sounds clear, SpO₂ 90%.
- **C**—Skin warm and flushed; pulse is strong and present radially at 75 bpm.

- **D**—Patient is awake but slightly confused. Patient cannot remember events leading to collision. GCS 11 (E3, V3, M5).
- **E**—Palpable implant to left upper chest.

The patient first wants to wait for his wife, but ultimately agrees to transport and further assessment. The patient is maintained with spinal motion restriction, placed on the stretcher, and then loaded into the ambulance.

Vital Signs:

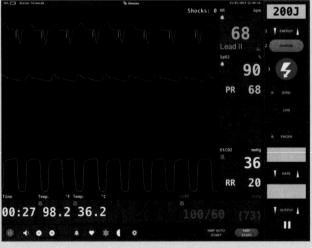

© National Association of Emergency Medical Technicians (NAEMT)

Secondary Assessment:

Detailed Physical Exam

HEENT:

Large hematoma to
the forehead with
bruising
Pupils 4 mm round
and reactive

Heart and Lungs:

Lungs clear bilaterally,
reddening to the
sternal area, no
deformity or crepitus,
palpable implant
resembling pacemaker
to left upper anterior
chest

Neuro:

Slightly confused but
alert and able to
communicate

Abdomen and Pelvis:

Abdomen soft,
nontender
Pelvis intact

Upper Extremities:

No obvious injury
noted

Lower Extremities:

No obvious injury
noted

© National Association of Emergency Medical Technicians (NAEMT)

Considering your transport decision, you reference the National Guidelines for the Field Triage of Injured Patients after your detailed assessment because you suspect your patient has sustained a TBI.

Questions:

- Does the patient need to be ventilated?
- Why does the patient have a normal heart rate with hypotension?

- What concerns are there with the chest wall findings?
- What does the finding of an implanted cardioverter defibrillator (ICD) imply?
- How do these findings complicate management of this patient?
- What indicators are present that the patient may have some type of TBI?
- Is identifying the specific type of TBI important?

Pathophysiology of Traumatic Brain Injury

Cerebral Blood Flow

It's critical that the brain's neurons receive a constant flow of blood to ensure a constant supply of oxygen and glucose. This constant cerebral blood flow is maintained by ensuring:

1. An adequate pressure (cerebral perfusion pressure) to force blood through the brain

2. A regulatory mechanism (autoregulation) that ensures constant blood flow by varying the resistance to blood flow as the perfusion pressure changes

Cerebral Perfusion Pressure

Cerebral perfusion pressure is the amount of pressure available to push blood through the cerebral circulation and maintain blood flow and oxygen and glucose delivery to the energy-demanding cells of the brain. Cerebral perfusion pressure relates directly to the patient's mean arterial pressure (MAP) and ICP. The

MAP is the average pressure in the arteries during one cardiac cycle and is an indicator of perfusion to vital organs.

Cerebral perfusion pressure is expressed by the following formula:

$$\text{Cerebral perfusion pressure} = \text{Mean arterial pressure} - \text{Intracranial pressure}$$

or

$$\text{CPP} = \text{MAP} - \text{ICP}$$

MAP Those Numbers

Normal MAP ranges from 85 to 95 mm Hg. In adults, ICP is normally below 15 mm Hg. It's usually 3 to 7 mm Hg in children and 1.5 to 6 mm Hg in infants. Therefore, cerebral perfusion pressure is normally about 70 to 80 mm Hg. Sudden increases or decreases in blood pressure and ICP may affect cerebral perfusion.

Although it is impossible to know what a patient's ICP is in the prehospital environment, it is vital to understand the importance of maintaining a normal blood pressure in the patient with a TBI.

The relationship among cerebral perfusion pressure, ICP, and MAP is important in trauma. Acute intracranial bleeding causes compression to surrounding tissues and an increased ICP. This is termed *mass effect*. As the ICP increases, the amount of pressure needed to push blood through the brain also increases. The MAP will increase to maintain CPP. If the MAP can't keep up with the increase in ICP or if treatment to decrease the ICP isn't started quickly, the amount of blood flowing through the brain decreases, leading to ischemic brain damage and impaired brain function. In the absence of an ICP monitor, the best practice is to maintain a high-normal MAP.

Hyperventilation, Blood Flow, and ICP

Hyperventilation has been used to reduce ICP but also adversely impacts cerebral blood flow. In fact, data suggest that hyperventilation more reliably reduces cerebral blood flow than ICP. Routine hyperventilation of a patient with a TBI is no longer recommended. Controlled hyperventilation should be reserved for patients expressing signs of brain herniation.

Pupillary Response

- Unequal pupils are an indicator of increased intracranial pressure.
- When ICP increases, it can compress the third cranial nerve, which crosses the surface of the tentorium cerebelli. This will cause the nerve's function to be impaired, causing dilation.
- Ongoing assessment of the patient's pupils is extremely important, looking for changes that may indicate worsening intracranial pressure.
- Caution! Do not look at the pupils during the primary survey and then not check them again throughout patient care and transport. It is not a one and done!

The Glasgow Coma Scale Classification of Traumatic Brain Injuries

- *Mild:* 13–15
- *Moderate:* 9–12
- *Severe:* 3–8

Glasgow Coma Scale

Establishing an *accurate* baseline Glasgow coma score (GCS) score early in the injury process is an extremely valuable resource that will help direct care long after the patient is handed off at the hospital. The GCS should be reported with a numeric value for each of the three components (**Figure 5A-8**). If a component of the GCS is not testable, it should be noted. Patients who are intubated cannot talk and receive a verbal score of 1T to indicate intubation.

The overall GCS score is good for comparison and tracking. When possible, identify the reason for a patient's altered state. For example, you assess blood glucose level (BGL) with all trauma patients, and you find your patient is in a state of hypoglycemia. Or, your patient has taken narcotics.

FOR MORE INFORMATION

Refer to the "Physiology" section of Chapter 8: Head and Neck Trauma in the PHTLS 10th edition main text.

Mass Effect and Herniation

The secondary injury mechanisms you'll see most often are those related to mass effect. They're the result of the complex interactions among the brain, CSF, and blood

Eye Opening	Points
Spontaneous eye opening	4
Eye opening on command	3
Eye opening to pressure	2
No eye opening	1
Best Verbal Response	
Answers appropriately (oriented)	5
Gives confused answers	4
Inappropriate words	3
Makes unintelligible noises	2
Makes no verbal response	1
Best Motor Response	
Follows command	6
Localizes	5
Normal flexion response	4
Abnormal flexion response	3
Extension response	2
Gives no motor response	1
Total	

Figure 5A-8 Glasgow Coma Scale (GCS).

© Jones & Bartlett Learning

against the skull, as described by the Monro-Kellie doctrine, discussed earlier.

In response to an expanding mass, the brain's first compensatory mechanism is to decrease the volume of intracranial CSF. The CSF circulates within and around the brain, brain stem, and spinal cord, but as the mass expands, CSF gets forced out of the head. Venous drainage also increases to help reduce blood volume inside the cranial vault. These two mechanisms prevent ICP from rising during the early phase of mass accumulation, and the patient may seem asymptomatic. As the mass size increases past the threshold of blood and CSF removal, ICP will start to increase rapidly. The effect of the mass is to shift the brain across and through fixed structures in the skull, eventually causing portions of the brain to herniate through or around some of them. This causes compression of the brain's most vital centers and jeopardizes their arterial blood supply.

The consequences of this movement toward and through the foramen magnum are described as the various herniation syndromes. These syndromes can occur in combination with each other.

Signs of Herniation

There are different types of clinical herniation syndromes. Clinical features of the herniating symptoms can help identify a patient who is herniating. Herniation signs progress as the herniation progresses.

Clinical Signs of Herniation

- Dilated or "blown" pupil on same side as herniation
- Loss of function of the motor tract resulting in weakness on the opposite side of the body and the Babinski reflex
  - *Babinski reflex*—stimulation of the lateral plantar aspect of the foot leads to extension (dorsiflexion or upward movement) of the big toe. Also, there may be fanning of the other toes.
  - Considered normal in infants and toddlers up to 24 months of age.
- Destruction of brainstem structures, which can result in abnormal posturing:
  - Decorticate (**Figure 5A-9A**)
    · Abnormal flexion of the upper extremities
    · Rigidity and extension of the lower extremities
    · Occurs with destruction of the red nucleus or the vestibular nuclei in the brain stem
  - Decerebrate (**Figure 5A-9B**)
    · More ominous than decorticate
    · All extremities extend
    · Arching of spine may occur
    · Occurs with injury and damage to brain stem
  - Coma
- *Cushing reflex*—triggered by tissue hypoxia and increased systolic BP
  - Can lead to Cushing triad:
    · Bradycardia
    · Hypertension
    · Alterations in ventilatory patterns (e.g., Cheyne-Stokes respirations)

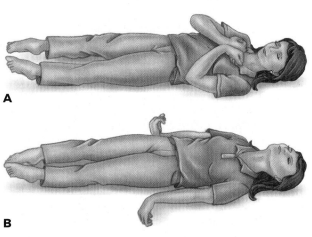

A

B

Figure 5A-9 **A.** Decorticate posturing. **B.** Decerebrate posturing.

© Jones & Bartlett Learning

Cushing Triad

Cushing triad describes the combination of findings that occur with increased ICP: bradycardia, increased blood pressure associated with a widened pulse pressure, and irregular respirations, such as Cheyne-Stokes breathing.

It Gets Worse

Herniation may lead to a terminal event where the extremities become flaccid and motor activity is absent.

FOR MORE INFORMATION

Refer to the "Pathophysiology of Traumatic Brain Injury: Secondary Brain Injury" section of Chapter 8: Head and Neck Trauma in the PHTLS 10th edition main text.

Treatment
Treatment Goals

Preventing secondary injury is the primary goal of the prehospital practitioner.

- Prevent hypoxia.
  - Provide supplemental oxygen to maintain O_2 saturation > 94%.
  - Perform continuous pulse oximetry.
- Support ventilations when needed.
  - Reserve controlled hyperventilation to 30 mm Hg for signs and symptoms of herniation as described.
- Prevent hypotension.
  - This patient has a marginal blood pressure and MAP and would probably benefit from fluid therapy, but the goal would be to prevent further drop in noninvasive blood pressure and maintain a systolic blood pressure > 110 mm Hg.
  - Support the patient's blood pressure with fluids.
  - Measure systolic and diastolic blood pressure frequently.
- Prevent hypothermia.
  - Normothermia is the goal for patients with TBI.
- Maintain $ETCO_2$ at 35 to 40 mm Hg.
  - $ETCO_2$ should be closely monitored and maintained within this specific range except for controlled hyperventilation in suspected herniation.
- Monitor blood glucose.
  - Hypo- and hyperglycemia can be very detrimental to the brain-injured patient.

- Check BGL at least once on all trauma patients in the prehospital environment.
- Target BGL in a brain-injured patient is 80 to 180 mg/dL.
- Often hypoglycemia is the causative event that leads to the trauma; for example, MVC or fall due to passing out from hypoglycemia with the patient sustaining trauma.
- Promote venous drainage of the head.
  - Ensure proper fit of cervical collar; a collar that is too tight reduces venous draining.

Transport

The 2021 National Guideline for the Field Triage of Injured Patients indicates that patients with moderate and severe TBI meet the Red criteria and should be transported to the highest level trauma center available within the geographic constraints of the regional trauma system. The trauma center should be able to perform CT imaging and provide prompt neurosurgical consultation and intervention (including ICP monitoring, if indicated).

Take a TBI Lying Down

In general, patients with TBI should be transported in a supine position because of the presence of other injuries. Although elevating the head on the ambulance stretcher or long backboard (reverse Trendelenburg position) may decrease ICP, cerebral perfusion pressure may be jeopardized, especially if the head is elevated higher than 30 degrees.

FOR MORE INFORMATION

Refer to the "Transport" section of Chapter 8: Head and Neck Trauma in the PHTLS 10th edition main text.

CASE STUDY: WRAP-UP

You arrive at the trauma center ventilating the patient via bag-mask device. The patient remains GCS 11. You give the patient report and care is transferred. The patient is diagnosed with a subdural hematoma and is taken to the operating room for emergent craniotomy.

After several days in the ICU postoperatively, he is transferred to a neuro bed with an improving prognosis. He is also diagnosed with a mild nondisplaced sternal fracture.

SUMMARY

- There are three things in the skull: brain matter, blood, and CSF; any of these outside of their "container" is catastrophic.

- Recognizing a TBI's potential existence based on mechanism and assessment is more important than identifying the type of TBI.

- Have a high index of suspicion with all blunt force trauma, even in the absence of obvious injury.

- Nothing can be done to reverse or fix the results of the primary injury; focus should be on mitigating the secondary injury.

- Maintain suspicion for the presence of a TBI, protect the airway, support BP, and ensure oxygenation—protect against hypoxia.

CASE STUDY RECAP

Dispatch	
Is the scene safe?	■ The fire department has secured the scene and advised you it is safe. ■ However, any scene can quickly become an unsafe one, so always maintain situational awareness for potential dangers, even on a "safe" scene.
How and where should you park your ambulance?	■ You should be parked between traffic and the scene to provide some form of shielding to the EMS crew. ■ Look at the power lines. You should park at least two power poles away from the scene to ensure safety from downed lines.
Is the power pole stable, and/or is there a threat of electrocution from power lines?	■ Even though the fire department has stated the scene is safe, we have a personal responsibility for our own safety and a quick scene survey is warranted.
Should the local power company be present?	■ Yes
How does the knowledge that the airbag has not deployed affect your approach?	■ An airbag that has not deployed after impact should be treated like a loaded gun and deactivated prior to working in or around a vehicle. ■ The negative cable at the battery should be cut/disconnected to remove power to the airbag charge prior to working in the vehicle. ■ Even after the negative cable has been removed, crews should operate with caution and take every step necessary to ensure the safety of the crew and patient. ■ Proper PPE should be worn by all on every MVC scene requiring extrication. This could range from reflective vest to full turnout gear. ■ Be sure to determine if the car battery is leaking.

What are the potential injuries to the patient?	■ The shearing force from deceleration alone is enough to cause intracerebral bleeding. High index of suspicion with speeds involved.
	■ Effects of deceleration on the heart and shearing energy created. Potential for aortic tear.
	■ Blunt force injury—head striking steering wheel causing trauma:
	  · Skull fractures
	  · Cerebral contusion (brain bruise)
	  · Intracerebral or intracranial hemorrhage
	■ Femurs fractured from knees striking dashboard.
	■ Pelvic ring from compression by femurs.

Initial Impression

Based on what you know, what kind of forces were exerted on the driver of the vehicle?	■ Blunt force with three impacts, and deceleration in a short period of time
What three impacts were involved?	■ Vehicle hits pole at potentially 45 mph (72.4 kph). ■ Driver strikes inside of vehicle compartment at potentially 45 mph (72.4 kph). ■ Driver's organs strike front of body cavity at potentially 45 mph (72.4 kph).

Primary Survey

Is there a need for hemorrhage control?	■ No, there is no obvious life-threatening external hemorrhage present.
Is airway management needed?	■ Not currently. Patient is talking and protecting own airway with adequate SpO_2 currently. ■ You must be prepared with a bag-mask device if his condition worsens.
Is spinal motion restriction indicated?	■ The patient has a mechanism that at a minimum would support manual in-line stabilization early in the assessment. ■ This patient would ultimately warrant spinal motion restriction.
Is the patient a reliable source for clearing the cervical spine?	■ The patient is slightly altered (confused) and there is potential for other injuries; thus, the patient is not a reliable reporter, and spinal injury should be assumed until proven otherwise.
What special considerations may be present for this patient?	■ Age—Refresh on atrophy of the brain in the elderly and how it contributes to traumatic brain injury. ■ Evidence of ICD and probable anticoagulants prevents normal physiologic response of the heart to trauma.
Could this patient have a traumatic brain injury?	■ Yes! In a patient with a suspected TBI, it is important to get as much information as possible about past medical history early in your assessment. The patient's condition may decline to the point of inability to provide this information in the future.

Detailed Assessment

Does the patient need to be ventilated?	■ Not at this point, but the prehospital practitioner should always be prepared to support ventilation.
Why does the patient have a normal heart rate with hypotension?	■ Unable to compensate due to fixed ICD
What concerns are there with the chest wall findings?	■ Patient possibly struck the steering wheel with no air bag deployment. ■ Could he have sustained a cardiac contusion?
What does the finding of an ICD imply?	■ Cardiac history ■ The patient could be on antiplatelet/anticoagulation therapy.

How do these findings complicate this patient?	▪ Patient could be at higher risk for intracerebral hemorrhage if on antiplatelet or anticoagulation therapy. ▪ Patient unable to have normal physiologic response to hypotension and pain.
What indicators are present that the patient may have some type of TBI?	▪ Mechanism of injury ▪ Physical exam with external signs of head trauma ▪ Decreasing GCS
Is identifying the specific type of TBI important?	▪ No
Transport and Ongoing Management	
What facility does this patient need to be transported to, and why?	▪ Closest available trauma center because this patient has signs and symptoms of a TBI with increased age, comorbidities, and the mechanism of injury

STUDY QUESTIONS

1. You're called out to an assisted living facility for a 72-year-old woman complaining of a severe headache and experiencing increased confusion. Staff reports she fell out of her wheelchair earlier in the week but didn't appear to be hurt; however, she's become increasingly disoriented over the last day or so. Vital signs show: BP 110/90; heart rate 118 and irregularly regular; ventilation rate 20 and slightly labored; SpO$_2$ 93% on room air. She is taking warfarin for a clotting issue. Which of the following should you suspect?
   A. Cerebral contusion
   B. Epidural hematoma
   C. Subarachnoid hemorrhage
   D. Subdural hematoma

2. Upon examination, you find the patient responsive to your presence, although she is clearly confused. Motor response shows reduced pain response but normal flexion. What's her GCS score?
   A. 15
   B. 12
   C. 10
   D. 8

3. What does the GCS score indicate?
   A. Mild TBI
   B. Moderate TBI
   C. Severe TBI
   D. No TBI

4. When you examine the patient's pupils, you notice the right one is dilated significantly and her motor response on the left is delayed. What does this suggest?
   A. Coup-countercoup injury
   B. Hyphema
   C. Hypoxia
   D. Uncal herniation

5. Which of the following signs would be most concerning at this point?
   A. A drop in systolic blood pressure to 88 mm Hg
   B. SpO$_2$ of 93%
   C. A field GCS motor score of 4
   D. Hemiplegia on the left side

6. According to the Monro-Kellie doctrine, what happens to the brain when it is still in a compensated state after a TBI?
   A. CSF, ICP, heart rate, and blood pressure are still within normal range.
   B. CSF increases, ICP decreases, heart rate increases, and blood pressure decreases.
   C. CSF and blood volume decrease, while heart rate and blood pressure are still within normal range.
   D. CSF decreases, ICP increases, heart rate decreases, and blood pressure increases.

ANSWER KEY

Question 1: D
The patient's age, use of a blood thinner, and the fact she fell recently point to a subdural hematoma.

Question 2: B
Eye opening: 4; verbal response: 4; motor response: 4 = 12

Question 3: B
A total GCS score of 13 to 15 likely indicates a mild TBI whereas a score of 9 to 12 is indicative of moderate TBI. A GCS score of 3 to 8 suggests severe TBI.

Question 4: D
When the medial portion of the temporal lobe (uncus) is pushed toward the tentorium and puts pressure on the brain stem, herniation compresses CN III, the motor tract, and the reticular activating system on the same side, resulting in a dilated or blown pupil on the same side, motor weakness on the opposite side, and respiratory dysfunction, progressing to coma.

Question 5: A
A systolic blood pressure of less than 90 mm Hg indicates secondary brain injury. Her SpO_2 is > 90%, and a motor score of 4 is not as concerning.

Question 6: C
In a compensated state, CSF and blood volume decrease, while heart rate and blood pressure are still within normal range.

REFERENCES AND FURTHER READING

National Association of Emergency Medical Technicians. *PHTLS: Prehospital Trauma Life Support.* 10th ed. Burlington, MA: Public Safety Group; 2023.

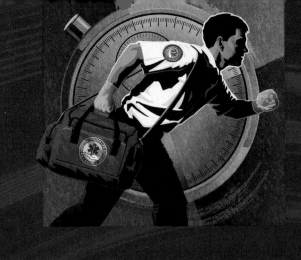

D—Disability: Spinal Injuries

LESSON OBJECTIVES
- Describe the pathophysiology of spinal injury.
- Recognize the signs and symptoms of spinal injury.
- Explain the rapid neurologic exam.
- Identify the indications for spinal motion restriction.
- Demonstrate evidence-based care for spinal injury.
- Identify special considerations in geriatric, pediatric, and other patient populations with spinal injuries.

Introduction

Traumatic spine injury (TSI) is potentially life threatening, and its severity depends on where the spine is injured and whether damage includes nearby structures, such as the spinal cord. TSI most often results from high-energy forces but may occur with a lower-energy mechanism of injury (MOI) in vulnerable populations such as older adults.

Causes of TSI include:

- Multivehicle collisions: 48%
- Falls: 21%
- Penetrating injuries: 15%
- Sports injuries: 14%
- Other: 2%

> ### QUICK TIP
>
> Injury to the components of the spine may not result in damage to the spinal cord; conversely, in some cases, the spinal cord, blood vessels, and nerves may be damaged without fracture or dislocation of the vertebrae.

If bony structures and supportive ligaments get damaged, it can lead to instability of the vertebral column, making the spinal cord and other nearby structures more susceptible to injury unless you restrict spinal motion. Immediate spinal cord damage occurs as a result of the trauma event, or primary injury. Secondary injury can be caused or worsened by motion from an injured spinal column. Failure to suspect, properly assess, and stabilize a patient with a potential spine injury can negatively affect outcomes. Prompt recognition and prehospital management of these injuries are important for timely stabilization in the critically injured patient, may guide future diagnostic and management decisions, and will reduce the risk of secondary injury.

> ### CASE STUDY: DISPATCH
>
> You are called to a local park on a warm and sunny day in early June. The temperature is 82°F (27°C). The patient is a 19-year-old female who was swimming with friends at a local river in the park and dove off some rocks into shallow water.
>
> Dispatch relays that friends pulled the patient out of the river when she didn't resurface. The patient is conscious, but cannot recall the details of what happened.
>
> **Questions:**
> - What is your initial impression of the case given the dispatch information?
> - What are your concerns about this patient?

The spinal cord can be injured at any level; the two main categories of SCI are complete and incomplete injury.

- *Complete SCI* affects both sides of the body and results in total loss of all function, including movement and sensation, below the level of the injury. Complete injury at the highest level in the cervical spine is catastrophic and often fatal before emergency personnel arrive on scene.
- *Incomplete injury* describes any SCI without complete loss of neurologic function. Movement, sensation, or both are preserved but may be asymmetric in a patient with an incomplete SCI. In general, physical dysfunction and long-term impairment increase the higher the injury, with a cervical spine injury being the most devastating. The loss of motor and sensory function after SCI can range from mild weakness to requiring a wheelchair or even a ventilator.

Understanding the limitations and potential complications of spinal immobilization are important in clinical decision making. The evolution in prehospital management of spinal trauma has led to the adoption of evidence-based protocols for spinal motion restriction and management that reduce the complications of immobilization using a rigid backboard, while at the same time limiting spinal motion in patients with an injured spine.

QUICK TIP

The initial management of a patient with suspected spinal trauma must include aggressive resuscitation and spinal motion restriction to prevent secondary injury and worsened neurologic decline.

Anatomy and Physiology of the Spine

The spine is a complex structure that:

- Facilitates movement in all three planes
- Disperses the forces from the head and trunk to the pelvis
- Shields the tenuous neurologic tissue of the spinal cord

Vertebral Column

The individual vertebrae of the spine are stacked in an S-shaped column, which allows multidirectional movement while giving maximum support. The spinal column is divided into five individual regions for reference. Beginning at the top and descending downward, these regions are the cervical, thoracic, lumbar, sacral, and coccygeal regions. Each vertebra supports increasing body weight as the vertebrae progress down the spinal column. Appropriately, the vertebrae from C3 to L5 become progressively larger to accommodate the increased weight and workload (**Figure 5B-1** and **Figure 5B-2**).

Spinal Cord Anatomy

The spinal cord itself consists of gray matter and white matter. The gray matter consists primarily of the neuronal cell bodies. The white matter contains the long myelinated axons that make up the anatomic spinal tracts and serve as the communication pathways for nerve impulses.

Spinal tracts are divided into two types: ascending and descending.

As the spinal cord continues to descend, pairs of nerves branch off at each vertebra and extend to the various parts of the body.

The spinal cord has 31 pairs of spinal nerves, named according to the level from which they arise. Each nerve has two roots (one dorsal and one ventral) on each side.

- The dorsal root carries information for sensory impulses.
- The ventral root carries motor impulse information.

Stimuli pass between the brain and each part of the body through the spinal cord and respective pairs of these nerves. As they branch from the spinal cord, these nerves pass through a notch in the inferior lateral side of the vertebra, behind the vertebral body, called the intervertebral foramen.

A dermatome is the sensory area on the skin surface innervated by a single dorsal root. Collectively, dermatomes allow the body areas to be mapped out for each spinal level (**Figure 5B-3**).

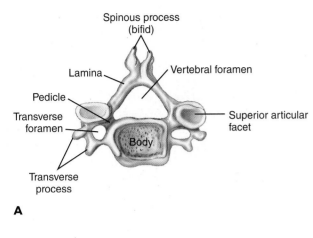

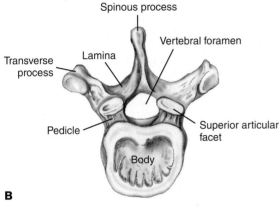

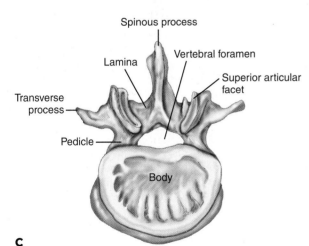

Figure 5B-1 The body (anterior portion) of each vertebra becomes larger and stronger in the lower spine because it must support increasing mass as it approaches the pelvis. **A.** Fifth cervical vertebra. **B.** Thoracic vertebra. **C.** Lumbar vertebra.

© National Association of Emergency Medical Technicians (NAEMT)

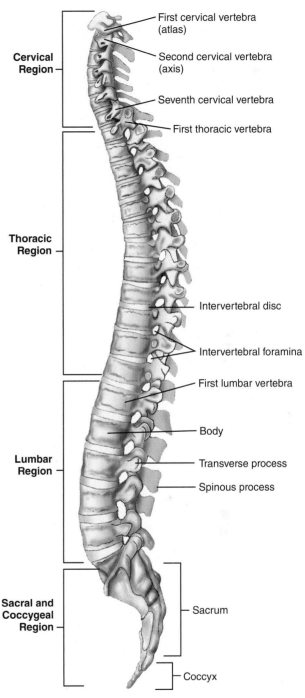

Figure 5B-2 The vertebral column is not a straight rod but a series of blocks that are stacked to allow for several bends or curves. At each of the curves, the spine is more vulnerable to fractures, hence the origin of the phrase "breaking the S in a fall."

© National Association of Emergency Medical Technicians (NAEMT)

The process of inhalation and exhalation requires chest movement and proper changes in the shape of the diaphragm. The intercostal muscles and accessory respiratory muscles like the trapezius also contribute to breathing. The diaphragm is innervated by the left and right phrenic nerves, which originate from the nerves in the spinal cord between levels C3 and C5. If the spinal cord is injured above the level of C3 or the phrenic nerves are cut, a patient will lose the ability

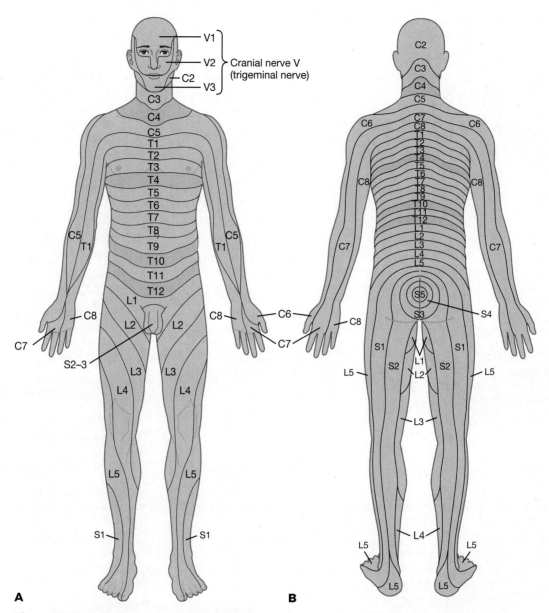

Figure 5B-3 Dermatome map showing the relationship between areas of touch sensation on the skin and the spinal nerves that correspond to these areas. Loss of sensation in a specific area may indicate injury to the corresponding spinal nerve or level of injury of the spinal cord. **A.** Frontal view. **B.** Posterior view.

© National Association of Emergency Medical Technicians (NAEMT)

to breathe spontaneously. A patient with this injury may asphyxiate before the arrival of emergency medical services (EMS) unless bystanders initiate rescue breathing.

QUICK TIP

It's critical to maintain control of the airway in a patient with suspected SCI. Positive-pressure ventilation may need to be continued during transport.

FOR MORE INFORMATION

Refer to the "Anatomy and Physiology" section of Chapter 9: Spinal Trauma in the PHTLS 10th edition main text.

Skeletal Injuries

Various types of injuries can occur to the spine, including compression fractures, burst fractures, subluxation, and discoligamentous injury. Although simple compression fractures are usually stable injuries, any of these injuries may result in immediate severe compression or (less commonly) transection of the spinal cord, resulting in irreversible injury. In some patients, however, damage to the vertebrae or ligaments results in an unstable spinal column injury but doesn't produce an immediate SCI. If the fragments in an unstable spine shift position, they may damage the spinal cord secondarily.

> **Spine Injury Deficits**
>
> A lack of neurologic deficit doesn't rule out a bony fracture or an unstable spine. Although the presence of good motor and sensory responses in the extremities indicates that the spinal cord is currently intact, it does not exclude a damaged vertebra or associated bony, ligamentous, or soft-tissue injury. The majority of patients with spine fractures have no neurologic deficit. A full assessment is required to determine the need for immobilization.

Spinal trauma can be caused by a wide range of mechanisms:

- *Axial loading* is a result of the spine being compressed, often from the head striking an object or a weighted object striking the head, sending the energy into the spine. Compression and axial loading also occur when a patient sustains a fall from a substantial height and lands in a standing position, transferring that energy up the spine.
- *Hyperflexion/hyperextension* is a result of excessive lateral bending, which happens in lateral and posterior impacts causing the spine to move sideways. This movement often results in dislocations and bony fractures.
- *Distraction* occurs when one part of the spine is stable, and the rest is in longitudinal motion. This pulling apart of the spine can easily cause stretching and tearing of the spinal cord.

> **QUICK TIP**
>
> Distraction-type TSI is a common mechanism in pediatric playground injuries, hangings, and certain types of motor vehicle crashes.

> **QUICK TIP**
>
> Determining the exact mode of failure of the spinal column is difficult because the injury mechanism is often the result of complex force patterns. Always assume that an injury severe enough to produce a fracture or neurologic injury has caused spinal instability until proven otherwise by further clinical and radiographic evaluation.

> **CASE STUDY: INITIAL IMPRESSION**
>
> The scene appears safe. The patient's friends are cooperative and answer all questions. None appears to be impaired by any substances, and you observe only towels and other swimming equipment on the shore of the river, along with plastic water bottles and snacks.
>
> There is no lifeguard. Bystanders report that the patient dove into the river and did not come up.
>
> The patient is lying supine on the bank of the river and is not moving. She is complaining of neck pain.
>
> **Questions:**
> - Is the scene safe?
> - What do you suspect the mechanism of injury to be?
> - Should manual spinal stabilization be done?

Spinal Cord Injuries

Primary injury occurs at the time of impact or force application and may cause spinal cord compression, direct SCI (usually from sharp, unstable bony fragments or projectiles), and interruption of spinal cord blood flow. Secondary injury occurs after the initial insult and can include swelling, ischemia, or movement of bony fragments.

- *Cord concussion* results from the temporary disruption of spinal cord functions distal to the injury.
- *Cord contusion* involves bruising or bleeding into the tissues of the spinal cord, which may also result in a temporary (and sometimes permanent) loss of spinal cord functions distal to the injury (spinal "shock"). Cord contusion is often caused by a penetrating type of injury or movement of bony fragments against the spinal cord.

- *Spinal shock* occurs for a variable amount of time after SCI (usually less than 48 hours), resulting in temporary loss of sensory and motor function, muscle flaccidity and paralysis, and loss of reflexes below the level of the SCI.
- *Cord compression* is pressure on the spinal cord caused by swelling of local tissues, but also may occur from traumatic disc rupture and bone fragments or development of a compressive hematoma. Cord compression may result in tissue ischemia and in some cases require surgical decompression to prevent a permanent loss of function, so prompt transport for imaging and definitive evaluation is important.
- *Cord laceration* occurs when spinal cord tissue is torn or cut. This type of injury usually results in irreversible neurologic injury.

Spinal Cord Transection: Complete or Incomplete

Spinal cord transection can be categorized as complete or incomplete.

- *Complete cord transection* occurs when all spinal tracts are interrupted and all spinal cord functions distal to the site are lost. Because of the additional effects of swelling, determination of the extent of loss of function may not be accurate until 24 hours after the injury. Most complete spinal cord transections result in either paraplegia or quadriplegia, depending on the level of the injury.
- *Incomplete cord transection* occurs when some tracts and motor/sensory functions remain intact. Prognosis for recovery is greater in these cases than with complete transection.
  - *Anterior cord syndrome* is typically a result of bony fragments or pressure on anterior spinal arteries resulting in infarction or damage to the anterior aspect of the spinal cord (**Figure 5B-4**). Symptoms include loss of motor function and pain, temperature, and light touch sensations. However, some light touch, motion, position, and vibration sensations are spared through the intact posterior column.
  - *Central cord syndrome* usually occurs with hyperextension of the cervical area, especially in patients who may have preexisting stenosis from degenerative or congenital etiologies (**Figure 5B-5**). Symptoms include weakness or paresthesias in the upper extremities but less significant loss of strength and sensation in the lower extremities. This syndrome causes varying degrees of bladder dysfunction.

- *Brown-Séquard syndrome* is caused by penetrating injury and involves hemitransection of the spinal cord, involving only one side of the spinal cord (**Figure 5B-6**). Symptoms include complete spinal cord damage and loss of function on the affected side (motor, vibration, motion, and position) with loss of pain and temperature sensation on the side opposite the injury.

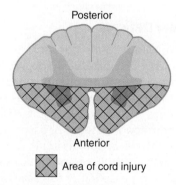

Figure 5B-4 Anterior cord syndrome.
© National Association of Emergency Medical Technicians (NAEMT)

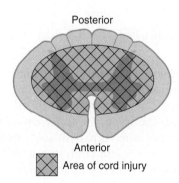

Figure 5B-5 Central cord syndrome.
© National Association of Emergency Medical Technicians (NAEMT)

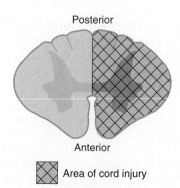

Figure 5B-6 Brown-Séquard syndrome.
© National Association of Emergency Medical Technicians (NAEMT)

Spinal Shock Versus Neurogenic Shock

Spinal shock represents a loss of motor and sensory signal transmission in the spinal cord as a result of injury. The severity of injury resulting from the contusion is related to the amount of bleeding into the spinal cord tissue. Damage to or disruption of the spinal blood supply can result in local cord tissue ischemia.

Neurogenic shock is a type of distributive shock caused by loss of sympathetic outflow to the heart and peripheral vessels. Without the right amount of sympathetic stimulation, unopposed parasympathetic transmission results in bradycardia and dilation of peripheral arteries and veins. Dilation of arteries results in loss of peripheral systemic vascular resistance, and dilation of veins results in venous pooling. This reduces cardiac preload—the venous return to the right side of the heart. In combination with bradycardia, a serious decrease in cardiac output may occur.

Patients in hypovolemic shock present with tachycardia in response to hypotension, and the skin is cool and clammy as the peripheral blood vessels constrict to shunt blood volume to vital organs in an attempt to maintain blood pressure. Conversely, the classic finding associated with spinal shock is "hypotensive bradycardia" that may require treatment with atropine (or another parasympathetic blocking agent) in addition to other methods of aggressive resuscitation.

Initial Resuscitation

Aggressive resuscitation plays a critical role in the prehospital management of SCI-related shock and in reducing neurologic problems and preventing the secondary neurologic damage that stems from loss of autoregulation. Early, aggressive volume and blood pressure augmentation can improve microcirculation and decrease the risk of secondary damage to the cord.

Ideally, initial resuscitation of the SCI patient should include measures to maintain a target mean arterial pressure (MAP) of 85 to 90 mm Hg for 7 days following the injury. This is often accomplished using crystalloids, colloids, or blood products through at least two large-bore intravenous catheters to restore as much neurologic blood flow as possible.

SCI and Hypotension

In a multisystem trauma SCI patient, it's important to weigh the potential risks and benefits of permissive hypotension. Given the risks of worsening SCI severity with transient low perfusion states, you should avoid permissive hypotension when SCI is suspected.

QUICK TIP

There is nothing you can do for the initial impact; however, using spinal motion restriction can prevent or reduce additional direct injury from disrupted vertebrae. Secondary injury can worsen the patient's outcome, but you can make a huge difference in patient outcome by recognizing and correcting secondary problems.

FOR MORE INFORMATION

Refer to the "Pathophysiology" section of Chapter 9: Spinal Trauma in the PHTLS 10th edition main text.

Assessment

Assess spinal injury in the context of other injuries and conditions present. After ensuring scene safety, the primary survey is the first priority. A rapid scene assessment and history of the event should determine if the possibility of a spinal injury exists, which would require immobilization. You should manually stabilize the patient with a suspected spinal injury in a neutral in-line position until you've assessed the need for continued spinal motion restriction.

Maintain the head in that position until the assessment reveals no indication for immobilization or the manual stabilization is replaced with a spinal motion restriction device, such as a cervical collar with a backboard, vacuum mattress, or vest-type device.

If the mechanism of injury is unclear, the scene assessment cannot be adequately performed, or available information is otherwise unreliable, assume the presence of spinal column injury and initiate external immobilization until you can perform a more thorough assessment.

Neurologic Examination

In the field, perform a rapid neurologic examination to identify obvious deficits potentially related to an SCI.

- Ask the patient to move their arms, hands, and legs, and note any inability to do so.
- Check the patient for the presence or absence of sensation, beginning at the shoulders and moving down the body to the feet.

Repeat the rapid neurologic examination after immobilizing the patient, any time the patient is moved, and upon arrival to the receiving facility. This will help identify any changes in patient condition that may have taken place after the primary survey.

QUICK TIP

You don't need to perform a complete neurologic examination in the prehospital setting, because it won't provide additional information that will affect decisions about prehospital care and serves only to expend precious time on scene and delay transport.

Using Mechanism of Injury to Assess SCI

Traditionally, prehospital care practitioners were taught that suspicion for a spinal injury is based solely on the MOI and that spinal immobilization is required for any patient with a suggestive MOI. Until recently, this generalization caused a lack of clear clinical guidelines for assessment of SCIs. MOI should never be the sole means of determining the need for spinal motion restriction, because it represents only one factor in a multifaceted decision-making process. Assessment of the neck and spine for spinal immobilization should also include assessment of the motor and sensory function, presence of pain or tenderness, and patient reliability as predictors of SCI. In addition, the patient may not complain of pain in the spinal column because of pain associated with a more distracting painful injury, such as a fractured femur.

Don't Get Distracted

The definition of what constitutes a distracting injury remains controversial; however, you should take associated injuries into consideration while assessing a patient for potential TSI and potentially lower the threshold for applying spinal motion restriction if a distracting injury exists.

Alcohol or drugs that the patient may have ingested as well as traumatic brain injury (TBI) may also blunt the patient's perception of pain and mask serious injury. Spinal motion restriction is not indicated in conscious patients with a reliable examination, no neurologic deficit, no neck or back pain, and no significant distracting injury. If any of these factors are positive on examination or are unreliable, continue spinal motion restriction.

Blunt Trauma

As a general guideline, presume the presence of spinal injury and a potentially unstable spine, perform manual stabilization of the cervical spine immediately, and assess the spine to determine the need for immobilization with:

- Any blunt mechanism that produced a violent impact on the head, neck, torso, or pelvis (e.g., assault, entrapment in a structural collapse)
- Events that produced sudden acceleration, deceleration, or lateral bending forces to the neck or torso (e.g., moderate- or high-speed motor vehicle crashes, pedestrians struck by vehicle, involvement in explosion)
- Any fall, especially in older adults
- Ejection or fall from any motorized or otherwise powered transportation device (e.g., scooters, skateboards, bicycles, motor vehicles, motorcycles, recreational vehicles)
- Any shallow-water incident (e.g., diving, body surfing)

Other situations often associated with spinal damage include:

- Head injuries with any alteration in level of consciousness
- Significant helmet damage
- Significant blunt injury to the torso
- Impacted or other deceleration fractures of the legs or hips
- Significant localized injuries to the area of the spinal column

These mechanisms of injury should dictate a thorough and complete examination to determine whether spinal motion restriction is indicated. If no indications are found, you can discontinue manual stabilization of the cervical spine.

Penetrating Trauma

Penetrating injury represents a special consideration regarding the potential for spinal trauma. In general, if a patient didn't sustain definite neurologic injury at the moment the penetrating trauma occurred, there is little concern for subsequent development of an SCI.

Penetrating Injuries

Penetrating injuries by themselves are not indications for spinal immobilization.

Numerous studies have shown that unstable spinal injuries rarely occur from penetrating trauma to the head, neck, or torso, and isolated penetrating injuries by themselves aren't indications for spinal motion restriction. Because of the very low risk of an unstable spinal injury and because the other injuries created by the penetrating trauma often require a higher priority in management, you should not immobilize patients with penetrating trauma.

QUICK TIP

Remember, the failure to suspect, properly assess, and stabilize a patient with a potential spine injury may produce a poor outcome!

Indications for Spinal Motion Restriction

The mechanism of injury can be used as an aid to determine indications for spinal immobilization (**Figure 5B-7**).

A complete physical assessment coupled with good clinical judgment will guide your decision making.

In 2018, the American College of Surgeons Committee on Trauma, the National Association of EMS Physicians, and the American College of Emergency Physicians updated recommendations regarding the use of spinal motion restriction. Based on these recommendations and current literature, spinal motion restriction should be considered when a blunt mechanism of injury exists with any of the following indications:

- *Midline spinal pain and/or tenderness:* This includes subjective pain or pain on movement, point tenderness, or guarding of the structures in the midline spinal area.
- *Altered level of consciousness or clinical intoxication:* For example, TBI or under the influence of alcohol or intoxicating substances.
- *Paralysis or focal neurologic signs and/or symptoms:* For example, numbness and/or motor weakness. This includes bilateral paralysis, partial paralysis, paresis (weakness), numbness, prickling or tingling, and neurogenic spinal shock below the level

CASE STUDY: DETAILED ASSESSMENT

Vital Signs:

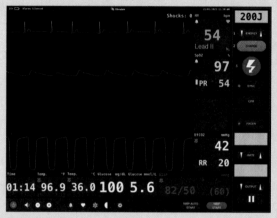

© National Association of Emergency Medical Technicians (NAEMT)

Secondary Assessment:

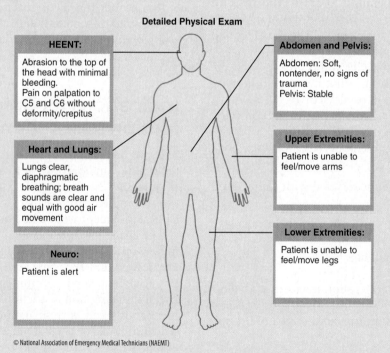

© National Association of Emergency Medical Technicians (NAEMT)

Detailed Physical Exam

HEENT:
Abrasion to the top of the head with minimal bleeding.
Pain on palpation to C5 and C6 without deformity/crepitus

Heart and Lungs:
Lungs clear, diaphragmatic breathing; breath sounds are clear and equal with good air movement

Neuro:
Patient is alert

Abdomen and Pelvis:
Abdomen: Soft, nontender, no signs of trauma
Pelvis: Stable

Upper Extremities:
Patient is unable to feel/move arms

Lower Extremities:
Patient is unable to feel/move legs

Questions:

- What pathologic processes explain the patient's presentation?

- Based on the patient's vital signs, what treatments are indicated?
- Is the patient at risk for hypothermia?

of the injury. A continuing erection of the penis (priapism) may be an additional indication of SCI.

- *Anatomic deformity of the spine:* This includes any deformity of the spine noted on physical examination of the patient.

- *Presence of a distracting injury:* This refers to an additional injury of such severity that the patient may be "distracted" from noticing spinal pain and report its absence (e.g., long-bone fracture or degloving injury).
- *Inability to communicate*

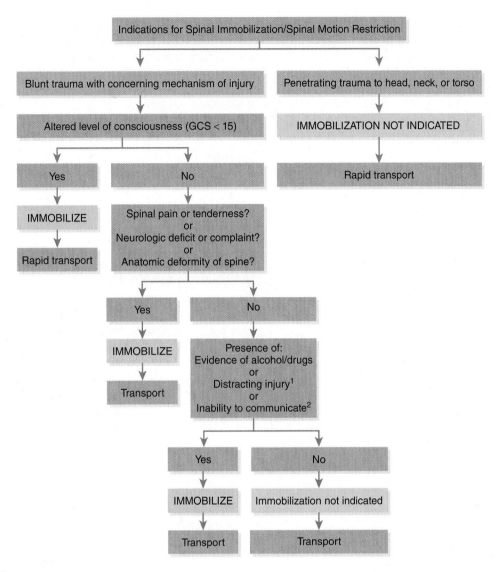

Notes:
[1]Distracting injury

    Any injury that may have the potential to impair the patient's ability to appreciate other injuries. Examples of distracting injuries include a) long bone fracture, b) a visceral injury requiring surgical consultation, c) a large laceration, degloving injury, or crush injury, d) large burns, or e) any other injury producing acute functional impairment.

    (Adapted from Hoffman JR, Wolfson AB, Todd K, Mower WR: Selective cervical spine radiography in blunt trauma: methodology of the National Emergency X-Radiography Utilization Study [NEXUS], *Ann Emerg Med*. 1998;461.)

[2]Inability to communicate

    Any patients who, for reasons not specified above, cannot clearly communicate so as to actively participate in their assessment. Examples: speech or hearing impaired, those who only speak a foreign language, and small children.

Figure 5B-7 Indications for spinal immobilization.

© National Association of Emergency Medical Technicians (NAEMT)

Several important signs and symptoms are concerning for serious spinal trauma; however, the absence of these signs does not definitively rule out spinal injury:

- Pain in the neck or back
- Pain on movement of the neck or back
- Pain on palpation of the posterior neck or midline of the back
- Deformity of the spinal column

- Guarding or splinting of the muscles of the neck or back
- Paralysis, paresis, numbness, or tingling in the legs or arms at any time after the incident
- Signs and symptoms of neurogenic shock
- Priapism

In an effort to reduce the unnecessary use of spinal motion restriction, particularly with a rigid long backboard, these professional bodies also recommend that immobilization on a backboard is not necessary if the patient meets all of the following criteria:

- Normal level of consciousness (GCS score of 15)
- No spine tenderness or anatomic abnormality
- No distracting injury
- No intoxication
- No neurologic findings or complaints

Your main focus is recognizing the indications for spinal motion restriction rather than attempting to clear the spine. Because many patients don't have a spinal injury, use a selective approach when performing spinal motion restriction, especially because spinal immobilization has been shown to produce negative effects in healthy volunteers, including increases in respiratory effort, skin ischemia, and pain. This selective approach is even more important with the older adult population, who may be more susceptible to skin breakdown and have underlying pulmonary disease. Focus on appropriate indications for performing spinal motion restriction but perform the intervention only if indicated to prevent associated complications. If no indications are present after a careful and thorough examination, there may be no need for spinal immobilization.

> ### QUICK TIP
>
> The cornerstone to proper spinal care is the same as with all trauma care: superior assessment with appropriate and timely treatment.

> ### FOR MORE INFORMATION
>
> *Refer to the "Assessment" section of Chapter 9: Spinal Trauma in the PHTLS 10th edition main text.*

Management

If you suspect TSI and spinal motion restriction is appropriate, prepare the patient for transport by safely limiting spinal motion. The goal of spinal immobilization is to limit spinal motion in patients who may have an unstable spinal column injury that could lead to secondary neurologic injury in the context of excess motion.

Fractures of one area of the spine are often associated with fractures of other spinal areas, so the traditional teaching has been that the entire weight-bearing spine (cervical, thoracic, lumbar, and sacral) is considered one entity, and the entire spine is immobilized and supported accordingly.

Patients usually present in one of four general postures:

- Sitting
- Semiprone
- Supine
- Standing

> ### Taking It Lying Down
>
> The supine position is the most stable position to ensure continued support during handling, carrying, and transporting a patient. It also provides the best access for further examination and additional resuscitation and management of a patient. When the patient is supine, the airway, mouth and nose, eyes, chest, and abdomen can be accessed simultaneously.

If you suspect spinal column injury, you'll need to protect and stabilize the patient's spine immediately and continuously. Techniques and equipment, such as manual stabilization, half-spine boards, immobilization vests, scoop stretchers, proper logroll methods, and rapid extrication with full manual stabilization, are interim techniques used to protect a patient's spine. These techniques allow for a patient's safe movement from the position in which they were found until full supine immobilization can be implemented.

> ### It's on You
>
> Although there's consensus about the general recommendations made here, current scientific research and understanding of spinal motion restriction is incomplete and imperfect. As evidence grows and recommendations continue to evolve, clinical management is ultimately the responsibility of each EMS practitioner, and you must understand local protocols and discuss the specific techniques to manage these patients with your supervisor and medical director.

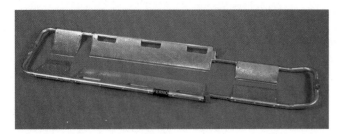

Figure 5B-8 Scoop stretcher.

© Jones & Bartlett Learning. Courtesy of MIEMSS.

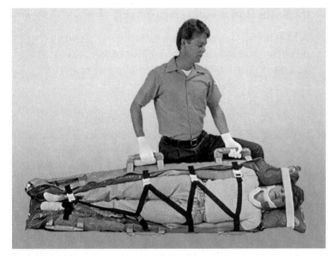

Figure 5B-9 Vacuum mattress splint.

Courtesy of Hartwell Medical.

There are a number of methods for performing spinal motion restriction. You can use a scoop stretcher (**Figure 5B-8**) or vacuum mattress (**Figure 5B-9**) as an alternative to a rigid long backboard, because they're often easier to apply and may be more comfortable. You need to immobilize the head, neck, torso, and pelvis in a neutral in-line position to prevent any further movement of an unstable spine.

In some instances, the patient may benefit from spinal precautions rather than complete spinal motion restriction. Spinal precautions can be performed by applying a rigid cervical collar and firmly securing the patient to the stretcher. This is likely more appropriate in:

- Patients who are ambulatory on the scene
- Patients who have mild to moderate neck pain, are reliable, have no neurologic deficit or complaints, and have no back or other thoracolumbar pain
- Patients for whom a backboard or other spinal restricting device is not otherwise indicated based on presence of distracting injury, decreased level of consciousness, or evidence of intoxication

Manual In-Line Stabilization of the Head

Once you've determined from the MOI that an injured spine may exist, the first step is to provide manual in-line stabilization. Grasp the patient's head, and carefully move it into a neutral in-line position unless contraindicated. A proper neutral in-line position is maintained without any significant traction on the head and neck. Maintain the head in the manually stabilized, neutral in-line position until you can complete mechanical immobilization of the torso and head or the examination reveals no need for spinal stabilization.

Contraindications

If careful movement of the head and neck into a neutral in-line position results in any of the following, stop the movement immediately:

- Resistance to movement
- Neck muscle spasm
- Increased pain
- Commencement or increase of a neurologic deficit, such as numbness, tingling, or loss of motor ability
- Compromise of the airway or ventilation

> ### QUICK TIP
>
> Don't attempt neutral in-line movement if a patient's injuries are so severe that the head presents with such misalignment that it no longer appears to extend from the midline of the shoulders. In these situations, the patient's head must be immobilized in the position in which it was initially found. Fortunately, such cases are rare.

Common Spinal Motion Restriction Mistakes

The most common stabilization errors include:

- Failing to adequately provide spinal motion restriction such that the torso can move significantly up or down on the board device or the head can still move excessively.
- Improperly sizing or improperly applying the cervical collar.
- Immobilizing the patient with the head hyperextended. The most common cause is a lack of appropriate padding behind the head.
- Securing the head before the torso or readjusting the torso straps after the head has been secured. This causes movement of the device relative to the

torso, which results in movement of the head and cervical spine.

- Inadequately padding. Failure to fill the voids under a patient can allow for inadvertent movement of the spine, resulting in additional injury as well as increased discomfort for the patient.
- Placing someone in spinal immobilization who does not meet immobilization criteria.
- Taking excessive time to achieve immobilization in the context of a physiologically unstable or potentially unstable patient.
- Using overly aggressive immobilization techniques that fail to prioritize maintaining and protecting airway integrity.

Complete spinal motion restriction is an uncomfortable experience for the patient. Spinal stabilization is a balance between the need to protect and immobilize the spine completely, the need to maintain and protect airway access, the need to expeditiously initiate transport, and the need to make it tolerable for the patient. That's why proper evaluation is indicated.

Spinal Motion Restriction in Special Populations

Obese/Bariatric Patients

With the increasing epidemic of obesity, care of the bariatric (overweight, obese) patient is becoming necessary more frequently. Transport of a 400-lb (182-kg) patient is becoming an all-too-common occurrence, and special bariatric transport cots have been developed for this purpose. However, when using lifting and extrication devices that are not designed specifically to accommodate bariatric patients, special care is needed to ensure that the safe operating limits are not exceeded. Also, additional personnel must be present to help lift and extricate bariatric patients to avoid causing further injury to the patient or prehospital care practitioners. This subgroup of trauma patients presents the challenge of balancing safe packaging and moving procedures against the short scene times normally recommended for critically injured trauma patients.

You should review your agency's spinal motion restriction (SMR) device's manufacturer weight ratings to ensure safe operation limits are maintained. Monitoring a bariatric patient's respiratory status when SMR is applied is also crucial. Placing bariatric patients supine can lead to respiratory distress or failure due to increased pressure on the diaphragm from excess adipose tissue.

QUICK TIP

Tongue obstruction, narrowing of airways, and chronic atelectasis create unique challenges for the supine bariatric patient. If full spinal precautions are initiated, ensure frequent airway assessments due to pathophysiologic changes to the structures of the airway and respiratory systems.

Be Safe: Use a Team Approach

When using backboards on bariatric trauma patients, you need to ensure not to exceed safe operating limits. Also, additional personnel must be present to help lift and extricate bariatric patients to avoid causing further injury to the patient or prehospital care practitioners.

Pregnant/Obstetric Patients

Some pregnant patients may require spinal motion restriction. Depending on the gestational age of the fetus, laying the patient supine may cause the gravid uterus to compress the inferior vena cava, resulting in a decreased blood pressure.

Securing a pregnant patient is performed using the same technique as for an average adult; practitioners should then tip the patient into a relative left lateral position, using blankets or padding for support, and thus move the uterus off the vena cava (**Figure 5B-10**).

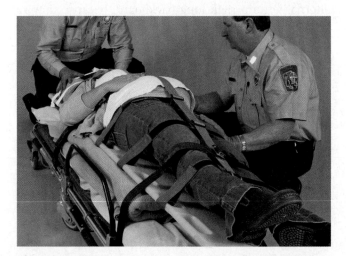

Figure 5B-10 Tipping a pregnant patient onto their left side helps displace the uterus from the inferior vena cava and improves blood return to the heart, thus restoring blood pressure.

Geriatric/Older Adult Patients

Geriatric/older adult patients can present with unique challenges. Curvatures of the spine, such as kyphosis, can make SMR difficult (**Figure 5B-11**). Patients with degenerative arthritis (osteoarthritis) of the cervical spine could experience a spinal cord injury from positioning and manipulating the neck when managing the airway, even if an injury is not present in the bony spine.

Less traditional means of SMR, such as a rolled towel and head block, can be used in the care of patients for whom a c-collar would not be appropriate; for example, a cervical collar might compress the airway and carotid arteries of a patient with severe kyphosis (**Figure 5B-12**).

A vacuum mattress is preferred over a longboard for older adult patients, because the mattress will mold to the patient's anatomy, reducing pressure points and providing appropriate support and greater comfort. Add a blanket or padding to relieve pressure to bony prominences when using a rigid longboard for spinal motion restriction.

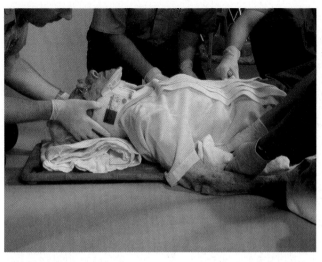

Figure 5B-12 Correct technique for achieving spinal motion restriction in a kyphotic patient when using a backboard. Padding is placed behind the head to fill the space that is formed as a result of the thoracic kyphotic deformity.

© Jones & Bartlett Learning

Patients unable to straighten their legs due to decreased range of motion should have additional padding provided under their legs for comfort and support during transport.

> ### Aging and Blunt Trauma
>
> Kyphosis (limiting c-spine range of motion), slower reaction times, polypharmacy, and changes in vision, strength, coordination, and balance predispose the geriatric patient to blunt trauma.

> ### Getting Old Is a Pain in the Back
>
> Osteoporosis, spinal stenosis, and spinal rigidity predispose the geriatric patient to spinal cord injury.

Pediatric Patients

Pediatric patients require consideration when using SMR. Although pediatric patients have the same indications as adults for SMR, growth and development will be critical in determining the appropriate SMR technique. EMS practitioners should maintain awareness of normal pediatric growth and development when determining SMR clearance in pediatrics. Follow your agency's guidelines for SMR clearance.

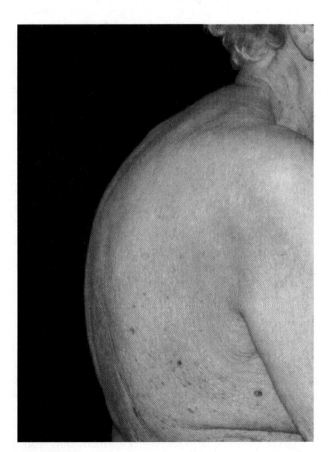

Figure 5B-11 Kyphosis.

© Dr. P. Marazzi/Science Source

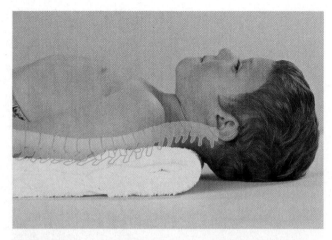

Figure 5B-13 Provide adequate padding under the child's torso, or use a spine board with a cut-out for the child's occiput.
© National Association of Emergency Medical Technicians (NAEMT)

Pediatric patients have a relatively large head size that varies by age, requiring EMS practitioners to make a special allowance for maintaining a neutral spine position in this population. Padding under the shoulders will maintain a neutral spine position (**Figure 5B-13**). Appropriately sized rigid cervical collars should be used to restrict any motion by following manufacturer's recommendations. Many commercial devices will provide sizes from infants to adults.

> **FOR MORE INFORMATION**
>
> *Refer to the "Management" section of Chapter 9: Spinal Trauma in the PHTLS 10th edition main text.*

Prolonged Transport

As with other injuries, the prolonged transport of patients with suspected or confirmed spine and spinal cord injuries presents special issues. Although backboards may be valuable for transfers over short distances or duration, they should not be used as stabilization devices for longer than 30 minutes. Such efforts should help reduce the risk for the development of pressure ulcers in a patient with SCI.

> **QUICK TIP**
>
> For transports that will exceed 30 minutes, consider using a scoop stretcher to carefully lift a patient, removing the long backboard, and then placing the patient down onto the ambulance cot.

You should pad any areas where there might be pressure on the patient's body, especially over bony prominences. Patients who are immobilized in a supine position are at risk for aspiration if they vomit. In the event the patient begins to vomit, immediately tip the backboard and patient onto the side. Keep suction near the patient's head so it's readily accessible if vomiting occurs. Insertion of a gastric tube (either nasogastric or orogastric), if allowed, and the judicious use of antiemetic medications may help reduce this risk.

Patients with high SCIs may have involvement of their diaphragm and accessory respiratory muscles, predisposing them to respiratory failure. Impending respiratory failure may be aggravated and hastened by straps placed across the trunk for spinal stabilization that further restrict respiration. Prior to initiating a prolonged transport, double-check that the patient's torso is secured at the shoulder girdle and at the pelvis and that any straps don't limit chest wall excursion.

> **When the Signs Are Low**
>
> Patients with high SCIs may experience hypotension from loss of sympathetic tone (neurogenic shock). Although these patients rarely suffer from widespread hypoperfusion, crystalloid boluses are usually sufficient to restore blood pressure to normal.

Another hallmark of a high cervical spine injury is bradycardia. If associated with significant hypotension, bradycardia may be treated with intermittent doses of atropine, 0.5 to 1 mg, administered intravenously.

Patients with spinal injuries may have significant back pain or pain from associated fractures. You can manage pain with small doses of intravenous narcotics titrated until pain is relieved. Narcotics may exaggerate the hypotension associated with neurogenic shock.

Patients with SCIs lose some ability to regulate body temperature, and this effect is more pronounced with injuries higher in the spinal cord. Keep in mind that these patients are sensitive to the development of hypothermia, especially when they're in a cold environment. Keep patients warm (normothermic), but remember that covering them with too many blankets may lead to hyperthermia.

All Level I and II trauma centers should be capable of managing the SCI and any associated injuries. Some facilities that specialize in the management of spine and spinal cord injuries may directly accept a patient who has suffered only an SCI (e.g., a shallow-water diving injury with no evidence of aspiration).

FOR MORE INFORMATION

Refer to the "Prolonged Transport" section of Chapter 9: Spinal Trauma in the PHTLS 10th edition main text.

CASE STUDY: TRANSPORT AND ONGOING MANAGEMENT

At this point, the patient has been packaged with spinal motion restriction and has an IV in place with a crystalloid solution at keep the vein open (KVO) after a 1-L bolus to maintain blood pressure. You reassess the patient throughout transport.

Ongoing Management:

- Maintain a patent airway.
  - The patient may require an advanced airway and pharmacologically assisted intubation.
- Titrate oxygen to maintain SpO_2 between 95% and 99%.
  - Hyperoxygenation can lead to the formation of free radicals, causing cellular damage.
- Titrate IV fluids to maintain a systolic BP of 90 mm Hg.
  - Use warm crystalloid solutions to prevent hypothermia.

- Use spinal motion restriction to prevent further secondary injury.
- Maintain normothermia.
  - Prevent shivering—warm the patient.
- Perform resuscitation measures to maintain a target mean arterial pressure (MAP) of at least 90 mm Hg to maintain spinal cord perfusion.
  - IV boluses of crystalloid solution

Note: Systemic hypotension (defined as a systolic blood pressure of less than 90 mm Hg acutely at any point following spinal cord injury) is associated with worsened neurologic outcome.

Questions:

- Where should you transport this patient?
- Could atropine be used for the bradycardia?

CASE STUDY: WRAP-UP

The patient was transported by ground ambulance to a Level I trauma center where she was stabilized. She underwent surgical intervention for a cervical spine fracture at C5 and C6, with no irreversible cord damage.

The patient was discharged several weeks later to a rehabilitation facility and discharged home 3 months later with limited mobility and will require further rehabilitation over time.

SUMMARY

- Spinal motion restriction should be determined by MOI and through a thorough patient examination.

- Stabilization should focus on appropriate treatment and reducing secondary injury to the spine.

- Neurogenic shock should be treated as appropriate to maintain good perfusion to the spinal cord to prevent further damage and a poor neurologic outcome.

CASE STUDY RECAP

Dispatch

What is your initial impression of the case given the dispatch information?	■ The incident may involve a traumatic brain injury and spinal injuries.
What are your concerns about this patient?	■ Because the patient was pulled from the water, airway and breathing should be concerns. ■ The patient is lying exposed and wet—hypothermia can be a concern.

Initial Impression

Is the scene safe?	■ Yes, the scene has been secured and no threats are found.
What do you suspect the mechanism of injury to be?	■ Blunt trauma from the patient striking her head on the bottom of the river, where there may be rocks, tree limbs, or other detritus
Should manual spinal stabilization be performed?	■ Yes, manual in-line stabilization should be performed given the mechanism of injury and patient's GCS motor score.

Primary Survey

Do you have any concerns about the results of the primary survey?	■ The GCS score; slow pulse; and warm, flushed skin
Do you suspect a traumatic spinal injury?	■ Yes, there is an abrasion at the forehead, suggesting significant force into the river bottom; there is no movement of the patient's limbs; she has neck pain; and her skin is warm with a thready pulse, suggesting compensated vasodilation—loss of nervous control of the blood vessels.

Detailed Assessment

What pathologic processes explain the patient's presentation?	■ The patient is at risk for and may be experiencing spinal shock. ■ Consider the patient's physical condition; that may explain low pulse and BP.
Based on the patient's vital signs, what treatments are indicated?	■ Spinal motion restriction ■ Insert an IV and administer a 1-L crystalloid bolus to maintain blood pressure, then continue with fluids at keep the vein open (KVO).
Is the patient at risk for hypothermia?	■ Even though the weather is warm and sunny with an outside temperature of 82°F (27°C), the temperature of the river water must be considered. ■ Removal of wet clothing will prevent the potential for hypothermia. Additionally, keeping the patient covered and exposing only for assessment will assist with achieving normothermia. ■ Normothermia must be maintained for optimal cell function.

Transport and Ongoing Management	
Where should you transport this patient?	■ Level I trauma center
Could atropine be used for the bradycardia?	■ Patients with high spinal cord injuries may experience hypotension from loss of sympathetic tone (neurogenic shock). Although these patients rarely suffer from widespread hypoperfusion of their tissues, crystalloid solution boluses are generally sufficient to restore their blood pressure to normal. Vasopressors are rarely, if ever, necessary to treat neurogenic shock.
	■ Another hallmark of a high cervical spine injury is bradycardia. If associated with significant hypotension, bradycardia may be treated with intermittent doses of atropine, 0.5 to 1 mg, administered intravenously.

STUDY QUESTIONS

1. You are responding to a call for 25-year-old, fit and healthy female who fell off a mountain bike. Upon arrival, you find the patient walking around. She is alert but complaining of pain in her clavicle and on her right side when she inhales. You notice that her helmet is split in two. What is the first thing you need to do?
   A. Complete a review of the ABCs.
   B. Check motor and sensory function.
   C. Perform manual in-line stabilization.
   D. Place her on a backboard.

2. During primary survey, you find the following:
   • LOC: alert and oriented; speaking in full sentences
   • GCS: 15
   • Airway: good air entry to bases
   • Breathing: bilateral
   • Circulation: skin warm, flushed, dry
   • Pulse rate: 112 bpm, strong and regular
   • BP: 90/42 mm Hg
   • Pain: Patient complains of severe pain at clavicle site and pain on inspiration at site of possible fractured ribs. No other injuries detected.
   What is your next step?
   A. Apply a cervical collar and in-line immobilization device.
   B. Treat for hypovolemic shock.
   C. Apply an arm sling for the clavicle injury.
   D. Administer pain medication.

3. When securing a patient to a backboard, which body part should you secure first?
   A. Head
   B. Torso
   C. Legs
   D. Pelvis

4. What type of padding should you provide for this patient?
   A. Use compressible padding under the shoulders and torso to prevent hyperflexion.
   B. Use firm padding between the back of the head and the backboard to prevent hyperextension.
   C. Do not use any padding. It can cause extension or flexion in the neck.
   D. No padding needed, but to avoid decreased venous return you should tip the backboard to a left lateral position.

5. While attempting to lay the patient supine for spinal motion restriction she becomes increasingly distressed and complains of shortness of breath and difficulty breathing. The fractured clavicle appears to move distally and increases the difficulty of breathing as the patient lies back. What should you do?
   A. Tip the backboard to a left lateral position.
   B. Raise the back of the stretcher.
   C. Let her sit up in a position of comfort.
   D. Administer morphine.

ANSWER KEY

Question 1: C
Because there's a possibility of spinal injury, you should bring the patient's head into a neutral in-line position.

Question 2: A
Although the patient's GCS is normal, she does have a distracting injury, and the state of her helmet indicates possible spinal compression/flexion, so you should immobilize the patient.

Question 3: B
When immobilizing a patient, you should secure the torso first, then the head, the legs, and the pelvis.

Question 4: B
Because the patient is an adult, you should use firm padding between the back of the head and the backboard to prevent hyperextension. You would pad a child's shoulder and torso to prevent hyperflexion, and you would tip the backboard for a pregnant patient to prevent decreased venous return.

Question 5: B
Because laying the patient supine increases the risk of airway/ventilation problems, raising the back of the stretcher slightly fundamentally maintains spinal alignment while reducing the ventilation issues.

REFERENCES AND FURTHER READING

National Association of Emergency Medical Technicians. *PHTLS: Prehospital Trauma Life Support*. 10th ed. Burlington, MA: Public Safety Group; 2023.

Sechrest R. Cervical Spine Anatomy (eOrthopod). https://www.youtube.com/watch?v=RNUpMNd_u1U. Accessed November 9, 2022.

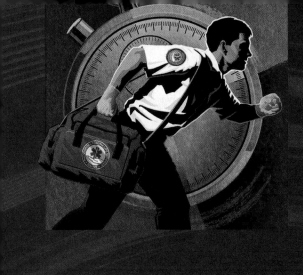

CHAPTER 6

E–Expose/Environment

LESSON OBJECTIVES

· Explain the critical value, risks, and benefits of exposing the patient during the trauma assessment.
· Describe strategies to maintain patient warmth.
· Recognize special considerations for pediatric, geriatric, and other patient populations during the trauma assessment.
· Explain the assessment and management of a patient with traumatic burn injuries.
· Identify unique factors affecting pediatric, geriatric, and other patient populations with traumatic burn injuries.

Introduction

This lesson has three sections. First, we highlight how exposing the patient is an essential part of the primary survey. Second, we review key environmental considerations for the injured patient. Third, we review the assessment and management of burn injuries.

Exposing the Injured Patient

Assessment is the cornerstone of all patient care. For the trauma patient, as for other critically ill patients, assessment is the foundation on which all management and transport decisions are based. An early step in the assessment process is to remove a patient's clothes because exposure of the trauma patient is critical to finding all injuries (**Figure 6-1**). Thoroughly exposing the patient is an important and yet often overlooked step of the primary survey.

The saying, "The one part of the body that is not exposed will be the most severely injured part," may not always be true, but it is true often enough to warrant a total body examination. How do you know you have found all injuries if you haven't exposed the patient? Think of exposure as a signal to you. Have you assessed XABCD, and have you begun

stabilizing all primary survey problems? After seeing the patient's entire body, the prehospital care practitioner can then cover the patient again to conserve body heat.

What Is Exposure?

Exposure involves many aspects. It is a:

- *Physical step:* Ensure all clothing is removed.
- *Consideration point:* Evaluate the impact of *environmental exposure* on the patient.
- *Decision point:* Articulate if you have determined the patient is critically injured and if you have a destination decision.
- *Transition point:* Shift toward the secondary assessment and assign responsibilities to team members.

QUICK TIP

Completely exposing the patient is your signal that you are ready to make a transport decision and begin the secondary assessment: vital signs, complete physical exam, and SAMPLER history.

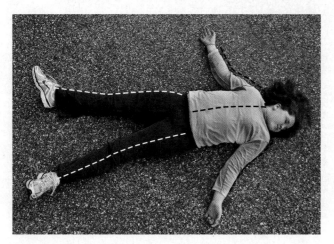

Figure 6-1 Clothing can be quickly removed by cutting as indicated by the dotted lines.
© National Association of Emergency Medical Technicians (NAEMT)

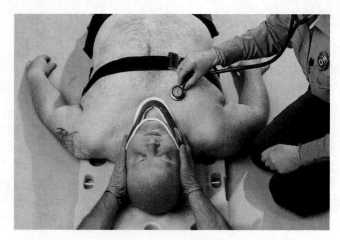

Figure 6-2 Exposing the patient allows for greater ease of visualizing all signs of injury.
© Jones & Bartlett Learning. Photographed by Darren Stahlman.

Risks of Incomplete Exposure

Leaving clothing on the patient results in not fully examining the patient. Incomplete assessments can result in missing problems that should have been discovered and addressed during the primary and/or secondary assessments. Causes for this worth mentioning are:

- Prehospital classrooms often verbalize removing clothing but rarely practice it.
- Concern about exposing the patient and embarrassing them (e.g., body habitus, exposing the breasts, etc.).
- Concern for what a patient may wear upon discharge.

Risks of Incomplete Exposure

- Failure to identify injuries
- Missing signs of patient deterioration
- Incomplete secondary and ongoing assessments
- Placing splints over clothing, leading to pressure sores
- Wet clothing worsening heat loss

We can overcome some of these concerns by immediately covering the patient and explaining to the patient why exposure is necessary. In some cases, leaving clothing on or under patients can lead to heat loss. It is easy to recognize soaking clothing such as when a patient is pulled out of the water. However, clothing may be damp from sweat, blood, or other fluids. Damp

clothing will pull heat out of the patient via conduction. Strategies for clothing removal will be discussed later in this chapter.

Advantages of Exposure

There are several advantages to exposing the patient. Besides the obvious ease of visualizing all injury signs, exposure helps to ensure that all damp and potentially contaminated materials have been removed from the patient, and ensures splints are not placed over clothing. Further, exposing the patient completely can serve as a physical cue for providers to ensure they have completed the primary survey, determined patient criticality, and assigned team member roles while transitioning to the secondary assessment (**Figure 6-2**). Finally, an exposed patient is an excellent reminder to apply blankets or other warming measures to the patient to prevent hypothermia.

QUICK TIP

Exposing the patient by removing clothing can lead to heat loss, hypothermia, patient anxiety, and embarrassment. Have strategies in place before exposing the patient to mitigate these risks.

No intervention is without risk, and removing the patient's clothing is certainly an intervention. Although the benefits generally outweigh the risks, it remains vital that practitioners consider and mitigate these risks.

Particularly when patients are laying on cold or wet ground, or when the ambient temperature is low, exposure can increase the risk of heat loss, which can make it more difficult for patients to compensate. You must also consider the location and any audience/witnesses when exposing the patient because this can become a source of anxiety and stress for the patient or any family members present.

Mitigate these risks by planning ahead. When reasonable, finish exposing the patient inside the ambulance and then immediately cover the patient with a sheet or blanket. Patients with burning or contaminated clothing may need to be exposed outside. In these situations, discretion is critical. Consider using a sheet to block the view of others and work quickly to ensure that the patient is covered as quickly as reasonably possible.

In many situations it will be possible to remove the patient's clothing without cutting it. When reasonable, loosen and remove clothing without cutting it. Even if the patient is stable enough to have their clothing taken off (rather than cut off), it still needs to be removed. Remember, removing clothing completes your assessment. It also saves the receiving hospital staff time.

Exposure Doesn't Mean Destroying Clothing

When feasible, undress the patient rather than cutting clothes. Be mindful of certain articles of clothing:

- Stuffed/down jackets (may make a mess).
- Leather outerwear (expensive).
- Unless absolutely necessary, consider leaving undergarments on the patient.

Often, only some of the patient's clothing must be cut; for example, a patient with a head injury might need their shirt cut but you can pull off their pants and shoes. When cutting clothing, your goal is to make as few cuts as necessary that will allow you to expose the body and remove the clothing. Undergarments can frequently be left in place. Remove them only when it is necessary to examine the genitalia, apply a pelvic binder, or place a Foley catheter. A bra should be removed when managing chest injuries.

Tips for Cutting Clothing

- Cut to expose *and* to remove clothing.
- Cut around a wound/fracture.
- Cut shoelaces instead of the shoe.
- Cut midline on the legs and abdomen/chest (see Figure 6-1 and **Figure 6-3**).

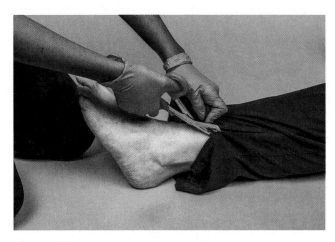

Figure 6-3 Expose the injury by cutting midline on the legs.
© Jones & Bartlett Learning

Isolated injuries require complete exposure of the injured area for thorough evaluation. When practical, assist in removing the clothing. Remove all of the clothing that you and the hospital will need to assess and manage the injury; for example, if a patient has a suspected broken lower leg, their pants will need to come off for a definitive splint or cast to be applied.

Note that there are special considerations for a suspected or known crime scene.

Exposure Special Considerations

- Isolated injuries
  - Single-system injuries must still be exposed to be fully evaluated.
  - At a minimum, remove the clothing necessary to assess *and* treat the injury in the field and at the hospital.
- Crime scenes
  - Patient clothing is considered evidence when a crime is suspected.
  - Avoid cutting through damage to clothing from penetrating objects (e.g., gunshot or stabbing wound).
  - When possible, avoid cutting through bloody or contaminated areas of clothing.
  - Protect potential evidence by placing it in a clean paper bag.

Temperature Regulation

As a reminder from the trauma triad of death, heat loss can lead to hypothermia, which worsens acidosis and coagulopathy (**Figure 6-4**). Humans lose heat to the environment whenever ambient temperatures are below 98.6°F (37°C). Applying blankets to the patient helps them maintain their own heat.

Inside the ambulance it is easy for practitioners to feel warm, especially while performing multiple tasks. However, it is important to resist making the ambulance comfortable for the crew; rather, it needs to be comfortable for the patient.

QUICK TIP

Remember the adage, "If we are comfortable, the patient is cold." This is why trauma bays at a hospital are kept extra warm.

Temperature Regulation

- Exposed patients are at increased risk of heat loss.
- Heat loss can lead to hypothermia, which is a component of the trauma triad of death.
- Ambient temperatures
  - Heat loss occurs via convection when ambient temperature is greater than 98.6°F (37°C).
- Ambulance cabin temperatures
  - Keep the cabin warm.
  - If you are comfortable, the patient is cold!

Risk Factors for Hypothermia

- *Age:* Older adults and pediatric patients have less effective thermoregulation; thus, they are more susceptible to hypothermia.
- *Alcohol consumption:* Ingesting alcohol causes vasodilation, increasing heat loss by radiation, and diminishes muscle tone, which decreases shivering.
- *Environment:* Immersion in water, cold weather, reduced wind chill, and so forth lower body temperature (**Figure 6-5**).
- *Medications:* Some medications can affect thermoregulation.
- *Mentation:* Patients with altered mentation, such as Alzheimer disease, may wander and get lost on cold days.
- *Physiology:* This includes impairments to thermoregulation, increased heat loss, and problems with heat production.

CRITICAL THINKING QUESTION

What is special about temperature in the human body?

- Cells work within a finite range of temperatures, nominally 98.6°F (37°C) ± 1°.

What happens if a patient becomes hypothermic?

- Hypothermia increases oxygen demand for the cells to maintain normothermia (such as shivering); it can also lead to acidosis and coagulopathy.

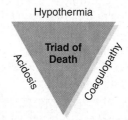

Figure 6-4 Triad of death.

© Jones & Bartlett Learning

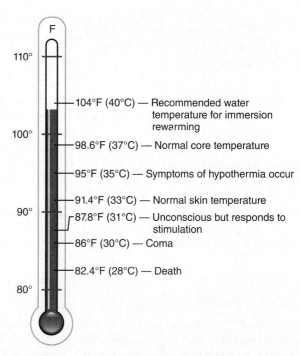

Figure 6-5 Symptoms of hypothermia occur at 95°F (35°C). The recommended water temperature for immersion rewarming is 104°F (40°C).

© Jones & Bartlett Learning

FOR MORE INFORMATION

Refer to the "Primary Survey" section of Chapter 6: Patient Assessment and Management and the "Burn Assessment: Expose/Environment" section of Chapter 13: Burn Injuries in the PHTLS 10th edition main text.

Special Populations

Both pediatric and geriatric patients require special consideration. Our thermoregulatory systems change throughout life and impact our ability to compensate and manage heat loss. With patients at the extremes of age, we use the same approach to our XABCDE primary survey but must make special considerations.

Pediatric Considerations

Pediatric patients have an immature thermoregulatory system. An increased surface area–to-mass ratio leads to increased heat loss through convection and conduction (**Figure 6-6**). Young bodies cannot shiver to

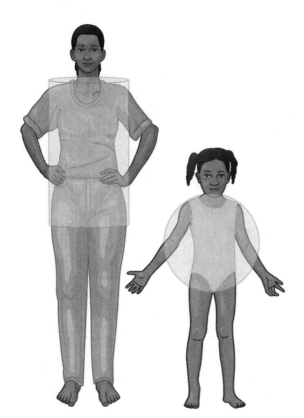

Figure 6-6 Children have a large volume-to-surface area ratio; the general shape of an adult is a cylinder, whereas children resemble a sphere.

© National Association of Emergency Medical Technicians (NAEMT)

produce heat. Be sure to place warm blankets under and over a pediatric patient.

Although exposure is critical and necessary to identify injuries, children may be frightened at attempts to remove their clothes. If the toddler or preschool child is not critically injured, a "toe-to-head" approach to the physical exam may be less frightening. Explain as you expose each area, and have a parent present whenever possible. Once the examination to identify injuries is complete, the child should be covered to preserve body heat and prevent further heat loss.

Older children, especially near the onset of puberty, may experience anxiety at having their clothing removed. Explain what you are doing before performing each action and continually during the assessment.

FOR MORE INFORMATION

Refer to the "Primary Survey" section of Chapter 6: Burn Injuries in the PHTLS 10th edition main text.

Geriatric Considerations

Older persons are more susceptible to ambient environmental changes. They have a reduced ability to respond to environmental temperature changes with impairments of both heat production and heat dissipation. Thermoregulation may be related to an imbalance of electrolytes, lower basal metabolic rate, decreased ability to shiver, arteriosclerosis, and/or the effects of drugs or alcohol. Hyperthermia may result from cerebrovascular accidents (strokes) or medications such as diuretics, antihistamines, and antiparkinsonian drugs. Hypothermia is often associated with decreased metabolism, reduced body fat, less efficient peripheral vasoconstriction, and poor nutrition (**Figure 6-7**).

As you expose the patient, you must also consider that older patients have weakened immune systems, placing them at increased risk for infection. This necessitates the earlier identification of all wounds for wound cleaning and dressing, and the prevention of pressure ulcers by avoiding pressure points while they lay on medical equipment and fabrics (**Figure 6-8**).

Weakened integumentary and cardiovascular systems can result in more superficial injuries such as skin tears and abrasions. Increased bruising can make it more difficult to determine if the patient's injuries are superficial or deep.

As you expose the older patient, pay particular attention to assess for medical alert tags and for medication patches. Older patients with memory difficulties

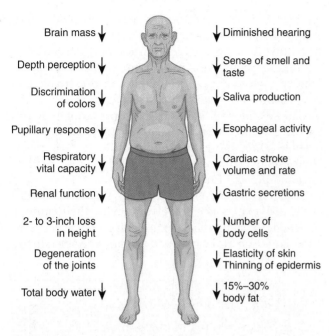

Brain mass ↓

Depth perception ↓

Discrimination of colors ↓

Pupillary response ↓

Respiratory vital capacity ↓

Renal function ↓

2- to 3-inch loss in height

Degeneration of the joints

Total body water ↓

↓ Diminished hearing

↓ Sense of smell and taste

↓ Saliva production

↓ Esophageal activity

↓ Cardiac stroke volume and rate

↓ Gastric secretions

↓ Number of body cells

↓ Elasticity of skin Thinning of epidermis

↓ 15%–30% body fat

Figure 6-7 Changes caused by aging.

© National Association of Emergency Medical Technicians (NAEMT)

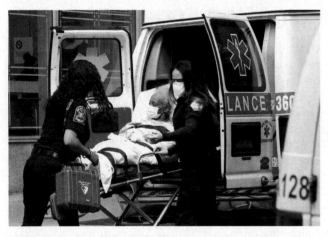

Figure 6-8 Remember that older patients are more susceptible to changes in the ambient environment and are likely to experience increased heat loss compared to younger adults at the same temperature.

© John Lamparski/NurPhoto SRL/Alamy Stock Photo

have been known to apply multiple patches without removing older ones first. Patches may need to be removed because medications may impair compensation.

Bariatric Patient Considerations

Obesity impacts all organ systems and poses many challenges for assessing and managing the injured patient. Specific to exposing the bariatric patient, providers must remain cognizant that these patients may be quite self-conscious about their weight, and exposing them may result in anxiety and emotional distress.

> **Obesity Is a Growing Problem in the Prehospital Environment**
>
> In March 2020, the Centers for Disease Control and Prevention (CDC) reported that the prevalence of obesity had increased from 30.5% to 41.9% in just over 3 years. During the same time period, rates of morbid obesity rose from 4.7% to 9.2%.

While exposing the bariatric patient, it is important to consider other environmental factors. Specialized prehospital care equipment may be necessary to safely move these patients. The typical EMS longboard is only 16 to 17 inches wide and was designed for adults with a normal body habitus. Stretchers are only slightly wider, around 24 inches.

Lifting nonambulatory injured patients can create a logistical challenge that must be addressed without embarrassing the patient or compromising expeditious care. Preplan rolling the patient onto an appropriate lifting system while removing their clothes. Pad any equipment carefully to prevent pressure ulcers, and package the patient so that you can continue to provide any required interventions. A team approach is necessary in order to avoid injuring the patient and the prehospital practitioner.

> **Bariatric Prehospital Considerations**
>
> - Over 40% of the U.S. population are considered obese; over 9% are morbidly obese.
> - Obesity makes examination difficult due to increased adipose tissue.
> - Bariatric patients may have increased self-consciousness.
> - You cannot rely on clothing to help support weight while moving a bariatric patient.
> - The patient is likely wider than a longboard, and may be wider than a stretcher.
> - Typical equipment may not fit appropriately.
> - They are at high risk for pressure ulcers.

Burns

This section shifts to another important topic: burn injuries. According to the CDC, in the United States, 1.1 million burn injuries occur annually, there is a fire-related mortality every 2 hours, and 50,000 burn patients are hospitalized annually. Postburn infections kill another 10,000 individuals annually (**Figure 6-9**).

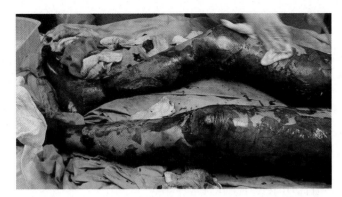

Figure 6-9 Example of deep, full-thickness burn with charring of the skin and visible thrombosis of blood vessels.
Courtesy of Dr. Jeffrey Guy.

CASE STUDY: DISPATCH

You and your partner work for an urban transporting EMS agency. You have been dispatched to a fire in an apartment building with a report of one patient.

It is 0410 on a Tuesday. Outside temperature is 18°F (–8°C). From the scene, you are 22 minutes away from a burn center and 12 minutes away from a Level II trauma center.

Question:

■ What possible injuries to the patient do you expect given the scenario?

Burn Assessment

Estimation of burn depth can be deceptively difficult for even the most experienced practitioners. Often, a burn that appears to be partial thickness can evolve to be full thickness. Or, in other cases, the surface of a burn may appear to be partial thickness at first glance, but later, after debridement in the hospital, the superficial epidermis separates, revealing a white, full-thickness burn eschar underneath. In the prehospital environment, estimation of burn depth, with the exception of clear full-thickness injuries, is even more challenging because the wound can evolve with the resuscitation needs of the patient. Often it is best to simply tell patients that the injury is either superficial or deep and that further evaluation is required to determine ultimate burn depth.

Superficial Burns

Superficial burns involve only the epidermis and are characterized as red and painful (**Figure 6-10**). These burns extend into the papillary dermis and characteristically do not form blisters. These wounds blanch with pressure, and blood flow to this area is increased

---

CASE STUDY: INITIAL IMPRESSION

You arrive on the scene of a two-story apartment building with a contained fire. Several fire engine and ladder companies, as well as numerous law enforcement officers, are on scene.

You are directed by the fire department incident commander to a corner of the parking lot, where you encounter a single adult patient who jumped from the building and is now covered by a blanket.

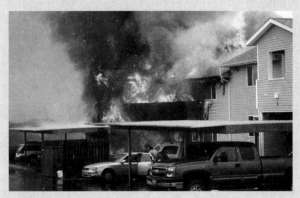

© LSqrd42/Shutterstock

■ First responders moved patient to a supine position and are holding manual c-spine.
■ Right lower ankle has obvious open fracture, and both lower extremities have deformity.
■ Visible burns to face and hands.
■ Patient is conscious.

Question:

■ What are your concerns for this patient?

---

compared to adjacent normal skin. Superficial dermal wounds usually heal within 2 to 3 weeks without scar formation. These wounds do not require surgical excision and grafting. Burns of this depth are not included when calculating the percentage of total body

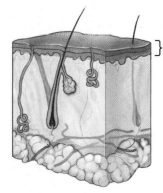

} Superficial thickness (first degree)

Sunburn

• Red
• Warm
• Painful

Figure 6-10 Superficial burn.
© National Association of Emergency Medical Technicians (NAEMT)

surface area (TBSA) that is burned or used for fluid administration.

Partial-Thickness Burns

Partial-thickness burns (second-degree burns) are those that involve the epidermis and varying portions of the underlying dermis (**Figure 6-11**). They can be further classified as either superficial or deep. Partial-thickness burns will appear as blisters or as denuded burned areas with a glistening or wet-appearing base. Superficial dermal burns extend into the papillary dermis. These wounds blanch with pressure, and the blood flow to the dermis is increased over that of normal skin due to vasodilation. These wounds are painful. Because remnants of the dermis survive, these burns can often heal, but generally take approximately 3 weeks to do so.

A deep partial-thickness burn involves destruction of most of the dermal layer, with few viable epidermal cells. Blisters do not generally form because the nonviable tissue is thick and adheres to underlying viable dermis (eschar). Blood flow is compromised, and it is often difficult to distinguish between a deep partial-thickness and full-thickness burn wound; however, the presence of sensation to touch indicates that the burn is a deep partial-thickness injury.

In partial-thickness burns, the zone of necrosis involves the entire epidermis and varying depths of the superficial dermis. A superficial partial-thickness burn will heal with vigilant wound care. Deep partial-thickness burns will often require surgery depending on their location, size, and patient factors; skin grafting can minimize scarring and limit functional deformities, particularly in areas such as the hands.

Blisters

In the prehospital setting, blisters should be left intact for transport. When blisters are debrided, the wounds are cleaned and antimicrobial dressings are applied; this cannot be accomplished well either in the field or during transport. Blisters that have already ruptured should be covered with a clean, dry dressing.

Full-Thickness Burns

Full-thickness burns are deep into the tissue and result in complete destruction of the epidermis and dermis, leaving no residual epidermal cells to repopulate the wound (**Figure 6-12**). They can result from prolonged contact with flame, liquid, or chemical elements.

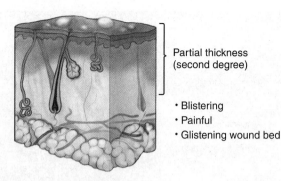

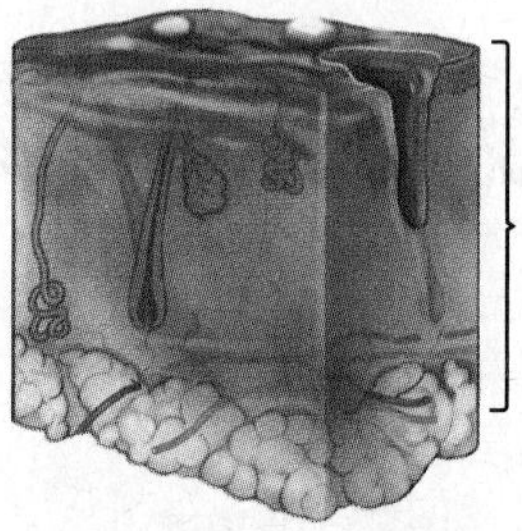

Partial thickness
(second degree)

- Blistering
- Painful
- Glistening wound bed

Figure 6-11 Partial-thickness burn.
© National Association of Emergency Medical Technicians (NAEMT)

Full thickness
(third degree)
- Leathery
- White to charred
- Dead tissue
- Victims will have pain from burned areas adjacent to the full-thickness burn.

Figure 6-12 Full-thickness burn.
© National Association of Emergency Medical Technicians (NAEMT)

Full-thickness burns may have several appearances. Most often these wounds will appear as thick, dry, white, leathery burns, regardless of the patient's race or skin color. This thick, leathery damaged skin is referred to as an eschar. In severe cases, the skin will have a charred appearance with visible thrombosis (clotting) of blood vessels (see Figure 6-9 earlier in the chapter).

Full-thickness burn eschar is insensate and will feel dry, thick, and leathery. Even though full-thickness burn areas are insensate, they are typically surrounded by areas of partial-thickness burns. Additionally, it can be challenging to distinguish (prior to showering the patient and cleaning the wounds) between deep partial-thickness and full-thickness wounds. Any wound that is not full thickness will cause the patient significant pain. Also, because full-thickness burns lose their tissue pliability, the patients can feel this constrictive effect, especially if the eschars (full-thickness burn wounds) are circumferential.

Circumferential full-thickness burn wounds around the thorax can be life threatening because they impede chest movement and ventilation. Similarly, full-thickness burn wounds around an extremity can lead to edema and compartment syndrome. Extremities with full-thickness wounds should be elevated as much as possible during transport to prevent additional edema. Full-thickness burns can be disabling and life threatening; patients with full-thickness burns should be managed at a burn center. Prompt surgical excision and intensive rehabilitation at a specialized center are required.

Prehospital Burn Pitfalls

- Becoming distracted by the burn injury and not recognizing and treating hemorrhage or other life-threatening injuries
- Overaggressive crystalloid resuscitation in patients with burns and hemorrhage
- Failing to recognize that the burn may not be the most life-threatening injury
- Failing to rule out hemorrhage in burn patients with hypotension
- Failing to prevent hypothermia
- Over- or underestimating burn size and over- or underresuscitating the patient

---

Subdermal Burns

Subdermal burns (fourth-degree burns) are those that not only burn all layers of the skin, but also burn underlying fat, muscles, bone, or internal organs (**Figure 6-13**). These burns are, in fact, full-thickness burns that also result in deep tissue damage. These burns can be extremely debilitating and disfiguring as a result of the damage done to the skin and underlying tissues and structures. Significant debridement of dead and devitalized tissue may result in extensive soft-tissue defects.

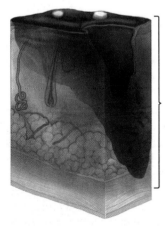

Fourth degree (full thickness with deep tissue damage)

Figure 6-13 Subdermal burn.
© National Association of Emergency Medical Technicians (NAEMT)

Burn Assessment

- Superficial (first degree)
  - Damages the epidermis
  - Red and painful
- Partial thickness (second degree)
  - Dermal layer damaged
  - Blisters present or popped
  - Most painful
- Full thickness (third degree)
  - Subcutaneous tissue damaged, including nerves.
  - Pain may not be present.
  - Skin takes on leathery appearance.
- Subdermal (fourth degree)
  - Charring present
  - Deep tissues exposed and burnt

FOR MORE INFORMATION

Refer to the "Burn Characteristics" section of Chapter 6: Burn Injuries in the PHTLS 10th edition main text.

Accidental and Nonaccidental Burns

Accidental burns are often caused by children spilling hot liquids and typically occur on the head, trunk, and palmar surfaces of the hands and/or feet. They are associated with irregular burning patterns from the splashing water.

Nonaccidental burns are a common source of child maltreatment. Burn patterns and anatomic sites are key clues as to whether a burn is accidental or nonaccidental. Clearly defined edges are often present on nonaccidental burns (e.g., a burn that leaves an imprint of the burning object such as a cigarette or an iron).

The most common form of burn seen in child abuse is secondary to forcible immersion. These injuries typically occur when an adult places a child in hot water, often as a punishment related to toilet training. Immersion scalds are often deep because of the prolonged skin exposure (although water temperature may not be as high as in other forms of burns). Factors that determine the severity of injury include age of the patient, temperature of the water, and duration of exposure.

The child may sustain deep partial- or full-thickness burns of the hands or feet in a glove-like or stocking-like pattern. Practitioners should be especially suspicious when the burns are symmetric and lack splash patterns (**Figure 6-14**). In cases of intentional scalding, the child

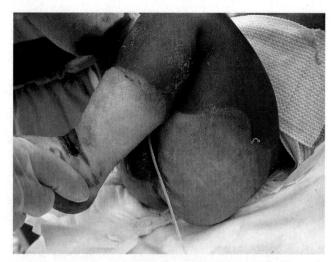

A

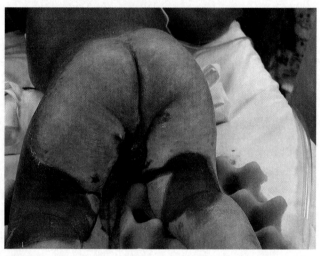

B

Figure 6-14 The straight lines of the burn pattern and absence of splash marks indicate that this burn is the result of abuse. **A.** Side view. **B.** Posterior view.

Courtesy of Dr. Jeffrey Guy.

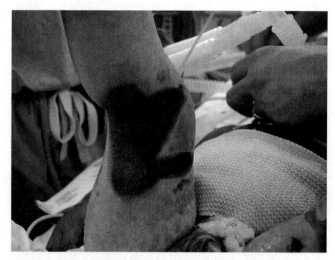

Figure 6-15 The sparing of the areas of flexion and the sharp lines of demarcation between burned and unburned skin indicate that this child was in a tightly flexed, defensive position before injury. Such a posture indicates that the scald is not accidental.

Courtesy of Dr. Jeffrey Guy.

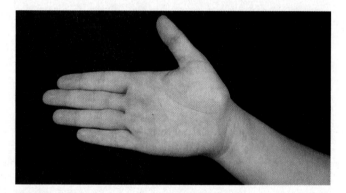

Figure 6-16 The rule of palms uses the patient's palm plus the fingers to estimate the size of smaller burns.

© Jones & Bartlett Learning. Photographed by Kimberly Potvin.

will tightly flex the arms and legs into a defensive posture because of fear or pain. The resultant burn pattern will spare the flexion creases of the popliteal fossa (knees) (**Figure 6-15**), the antecubital fossa (elbows), and the groin. Sharp lines of demarcation will also be seen between burned and unburned tissue, essentially indicating a dip.

FOR MORE INFORMATION

Refer to the "Child Abuse" section of Chapter 6: Burn Injuries in the PHTLS 10th edition main text.

Estimating Burn Area

A careful evaluation of burn wounds is conducted once the primary and secondary surveys are complete. At this time, the wounds are cleansed and assessed. Estimation of burn size is necessary to resuscitate the patient appropriately and prevent the complications associated with hypovolemic shock from burn injury. Burn size determination is also used as a tool for stratifying injury severity and triage.

The two most widely used burn estimation tools are the palmar method and rule of nines. The use of the patient's palm has been a widely accepted and long-standing practice for estimating the size of smaller burns (**Figure 6-16**); however, there has not been uniform acceptance of what defines a palm and how large it is. The average area of the palm alone (not including the extended fingers) is 0.5% TBSA in males and 0.4% in females. Including the palmar aspect of all five extended digits along with the palm increases the area to 0.8% TBSA for males and 0.7% TBSA for females.

Aside from gender differences of palm size, the size of the palm also varies with body weight of the patient. As the patient's body mass index (BMI) increases, the total skin surface area of the body increases, and the TBSA percentage of the palm decreases. In most cases, the palm plus the fingers of the patient can be grossly estimated to be approximately 1% of the patient's TBSA.

The most widely applied method is the rule of nines, which applies the principle that major regions of the body in adults are considered to be 9% of the total body surface area (**Figure 6-17**). The perineum, or genital area, represents 1%.

> ## QUICK TIP
>
> Practitioners tend to overestimate burn area and severity in the prehospital setting. Initial estimation is important for calculating fluid needs.

> ## FOR MORE INFORMATION
>
> *Refer to the "Burn Assessment" section of Chapter 6: Burn Injuries in the PHTLS 10th edition main text.*

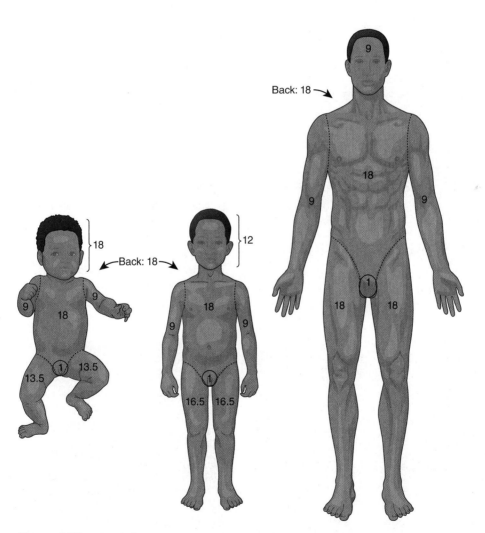

Figure 6-17 Rule of nines.
© Jones & Bartlett Learning

Critical Burns

Critical burns are extremely dangerous. Certain burn locations and types place the victim at high risk for complications, such as impaired ventilation, impaired perfusion, and infection. The presence of burns, particularly partial thickness or greater, to the following areas necessitates evaluation at a burn center:

- Hands and feet (**Figure 6-18**)
- Circumferential (**Figure 6-19**)
- Face and airway (inhalation burns)
- Genitalia

CASE STUDY: PRIMARY SURVEY

- **X**—No major external hemorrhage; some bleeding from open fracture
- **A**—Patent
- **B**—28, normal depth and rate
- **C**—100, strong radial pulses; skin is pale, diaphoretic
- **D**—GCS 15 (E4, V5, M6)
- **E**—Burns to both arms and hands, anterior chest, and face; open fracture to right ankle

Questions:

- What are the life threats with this patient?
- Is airway management indicated?
- What critical actions should you take?
- What is the estimated body surface area involved?

Stopping the Burning Process

The first step in the care of a patient with burn injury is to stop the burning process. The most effective and appropriate method of terminating the burning is irrigation with copious volumes of room-temperature water. The application of ice will stop the burning and provide analgesia, but it will also stimulate local vasoconstriction, which risks increasing the extent of tissue damage in the zone of stasis. Remove all clothing and jewelry; these items maintain residual heat and will continue to burn the patient. In addition, jewelry may constrict digits or extremities as the tissues begin to swell. Clothing items that have burned and melted onto the skin should not be removed but should be cooled with room-temperature water.

To effectively dress a recent burn, sterile, nonadherent dressings are applied, and the area is covered with a clean, dry sheet. If a sheet is not readily available, substitute a sterile surgical gown, drapes, towels, or a Mylar rescue blanket. The dressing will prevent ongoing environmental contamination while helping to prevent the patient from experiencing pain from air flowing over the exposed nerve endings. Airflow or any contact or movement of burned skin will cause a significant amount of pain for the patient. There has to be a balance with stopping the burning process and preventing air movement/contamination of the burn wound. Certain commercial dressings with sterile hydrogels can be used for both processes and may be beneficial in the prehospital environment.

QUICK TIP

Cover burns with a dry sterile dressing with nonadherent bandages. Do *not* use wet dressings or topical burn creams/ointments because these will worsen heat loss and can increase the risk of infection. Leave blisters intact and cover them with a dry sterile dressing.

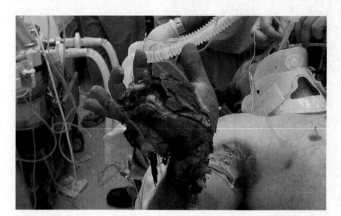

Figure 6-18 Patient after electrical injury from high-tension wires.
Courtesy of Dr. Jeffrey Guy.

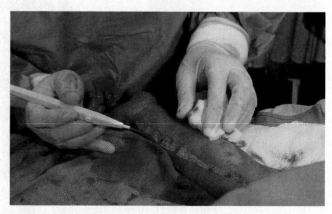

Figure 6-19 Escharotomies are performed to release the constricting effect of circumferential burns.
Courtesy of Dr. Jeffrey Guy.

CASE STUDY: DETAILED ASSESSMENT

Vital Signs:

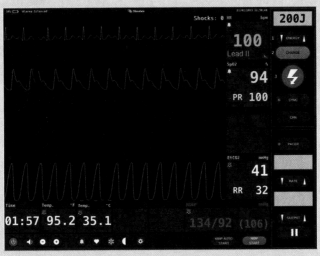

© National Association of Emergency Medical Technicians (NAEMT)

Secondary Assessment:

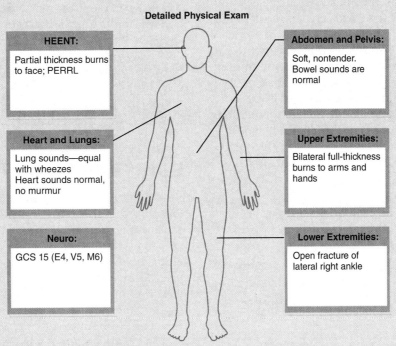

Detailed Physical Exam

HEENT:
Partial thickness burns to face; PERRL

Heart and Lungs:
Lung sounds—equal with wheezes
Heart sounds normal, no murmur

Neuro:
GCS 15 (E4, V5, M6)

Abdomen and Pelvis:
Soft, nontender. Bowel sounds are normal

Upper Extremities:
Bilateral full-thickness burns to arms and hands

Lower Extremities:
Open fracture of lateral right ankle

© National Association of Emergency Medical Technicians (NAEMT)

Primary Survey Reassessment:

- **X**—No hemorrhage
- **A**—Patent, supplemental O_2 via nasal cannula
- **B**—32, wheezes
- **C**—100, strong radial pulses; skin pale and diaphoretic
- **D**—GCS 15 (E4, V5, M6)
- **E**—Burns to both arms and hands, anterior chest, and face; open fracture to right ankle now splinted

Prehospital care practitioners have often been unsatisfied and frustrated with the simple application of sterile sheets to a burn; however, topical ointments and conventional topical antibiotics should not be applied because they prevent a direct inspection of the burn. Such topical ointments and antibiotics are removed on admission to the burn center to allow direct visualization of the burn and determination of burn severity.

Burn Care Considerations

After the initial burn care, there are many additional burn management considerations. Patients with large burn injuries have had their thermoregulatory mechanisms impaired. These patients are at high risk for excessive heat loss and hypothermia. Most patients arrive at burn centers cold! Be sure to cover burn patients with warm blankets and increase the temperature of the patient compartment in the ambulance.

Fluid loss will occur as serosanguinous fluid continuously leaks from damaged capillaries into the dry dressings. The larger the burn area, the greater the fluid loss. In addition, as open burn wounds weep and leak fluid, evaporation further exacerbates the patient's body heat loss.

Inflammation is the body's natural response to injury, and over the course of several hours the injured patient will experience significant third spacing of fluid as inflammation occurs in response to the burns.

Significant pain occurs from both exposed free nerve endings when the epidermis is burned, exposing the dermal layer, and the pressure within the tissues that worsens as inflammation develops.

QUICK TIP

Skip the antibiotics. Although there is an increased risk of infection following burns, there is no evidence supporting the routine use of antibiotic prophylaxis in the prehospital setting.

Burn Care Considerations

- Prevent temperature loss.
  - Cover patient with warm blankets.
  - Increase cabin temperatures above normal.

- Anticipate fluid loss.
  - Serosanguinous fluid lost from damaged capillaries.
  - Monitor dressings and change as necessary.
- Inflammation will occur.
- Pain can be severe.
  - Exposed free nerve endings
- Infection risk—but do not use antibiotic prophylaxis.

The Higher the Age, the Higher the Mortality Rate

Patients age 60 years and older have higher mortality rates for every category of burn severity. Older patients are also more likely to face complications related to burn injuries and subsequent hospitalizations. The top complications include pneumonia, urinary tract infection, and respiratory failure. Unlike in younger patient populations, those age 60 years and older have a greater mortality rate with significantly smaller burn size. In patients ages 60 to 69 years, mortality exceeds 50% at 40% TBSA; for those ages 70 to 79 years, mortality exceeds 50% at 30% TBSA; and for patients 80 years and older, mortality exceeds 50% at 20% TBSA.

Burn Fluid Resuscitation

Burn injury results in direct disruption of cellular integrity and ongoing release of inflammatory mediators, causing vascular permeability and an increase in microvascular hydrostatic pressure. This drives the large efflux of fluid from the intravascular space into the interstitium. The underlying goal of early initial fluid resuscitation is to replace the intravascular volume and support the patient through the hypovolemia in the first 24 to 48 hours.

The resuscitation of a patient with a burn injury is aimed not only at the restoration of the loss of intravascular volume, but also at the replacement of anticipated intravascular losses at a rate that mimics those losses as they occur. In trauma patients, the prehospital care practitioner is replacing the volume that the patient has already lost from hemorrhage from an open fracture or bleeding viscera. In contrast, when treating

Resuscitating a Patient with a Burn Injury

Resuscitating a patient with a burn injury can be compared to filling a leaking bucket. The bucket is leaking water at a constant rate. The bucket has a line drawn inside near the top. The objective is to keep the water level at the line. Initially the water depth will be low. The longer the bucket has been unattended, the lower the water level will be and the greater the amount of fluid that needs to be replaced. The container will continue to leak, so once the bucket has been filled to an appropriate level, water will need to be continuously added at a constant rate to maintain the desired level.

The longer the patient with a burn injury is not resuscitated or remains underresuscitated, the more hypovolemic the patient becomes. Therefore, greater amounts of fluids are required to establish a "level" of homeostasis. Once the patient has been resuscitated, the vascular space continues to leak in the same manner as the bucket. To maintain equilibrium with this homeostatic point, additional fluids need to be provided to replace the ongoing losses. It is important to keep track of the fluid that is being administered because overresuscitation can be as harmful as underresuscitation. In patients with transport times longer than 1 hour, communication with the receiving center should occur regarding the fluid resuscitation plan.

Some centers are starting to use plasma for burn resuscitation; as this practice gets adopted more widely, it may migrate to the prehospital environment.

the patient with a burn injury, the objective is to calculate and replace the fluids that the patient has already lost as well as replace the patient's anticipated losses over the first 24 hours after the burn injury. Early fluid resuscitation is aimed at preventing progression of patients to burn shock.

Maintaining urine output is essential in burn patients and is the primary indicator of adequate resuscitation. Patients with a > 20% TBSA burn should have their urine output monitored closely, and all patients with > 40% TBSA burn should have a urinary catheter placed to monitory hourly urine output. Burn resuscitation can be guided by urine

output, and the formulas presented in this chapter are aimed at restoring intravascular volume, which can be monitored by average hourly urine output. A challenge to using urine output as a goal for fluid resuscitation is when patients with extensive burns have sufficient shock to result in acute kidney injury and anuria; other endpoints of resuscitation, such as lactate and base deficit, will then need to be closely monitored.

Volume Resuscitation Calculation Options

- Parkland Formula
- Rule of Ten
- Pediatrics

The Parkland Formula

The amount of fluids administered for patients with deep partial and full thickness burns involving > 20% body surface area (BSA) should begin with 4 ml of lactated Ringer solution × patient's weight in kg × % total body surface area (TBSA). Fluid is titrated based on adequacy of the urine output. Avoid fluid boluses unless the patient is hypotensive.

The fluid resuscitation volume would be calculated as follows using the Parkland formula:

$$\text{24-hour fluid total} = 4 \text{ ml/kg} \times \text{weight in kg} \times \% \text{ TBSA burned}$$

$$= 4 \text{ ml/kg} \times 80 \text{ kg} \times 30\% \text{ TBSA burned}$$

$$= 9{,}600 \text{ ml}$$

Note that in this formula, the units of kilograms and percentage cancel out so that only ml is left, thus making the calculation $4 \text{ ml} \times 80 \times 30 = 9{,}600 \text{ ml}$. Once the 24-hour total is calculated, divide that number by 2:

$$\text{Amount of fluid to be given from time of injury to hour 8} = 9{,}600 \text{ ml} / 2 = 4{,}800 \text{ ml}$$

To determine the hourly rate for the first 8 hours, divide this total by 8:

$$\text{Fluid rate for the first 8 hours} = 4{,}800 \text{ ml} / 8 \text{ hours} = 600 \text{ ml/hr}$$

The fluid requirement for the next period (hours 8 to 24) is calculated as follows:

$$\text{Amount of fluid to be given from hours 8 to 24} = 9{,}600 \text{ ml} / 2 = 4{,}800 \text{ ml}$$

To determine the hourly rate for the final 16 hours, divide this total by 16:

Fluid rate for final 16 hours = 4,800 ml / 16 hours = 300 ml/hr

In general, lactated Ringer solution is preferred over normal saline. Normal saline has a lower pH of 5.5, is not electrolyte neutral, and large volumes can trigger a hyperchloremic metabolic acidosis.

CRITICAL THINKING QUESTION

How is fluid resuscitation modified for pediatric patients?

- Resuscitate pediatric patients using 3 ml/kg/% TBSA.

Rule of Ten for Burn Resuscitation

- Researchers from the U.S. Army Institute of Surgical Research developed the Rule of Ten to aid in initial fluid resuscitation.
- The percentage of body surface area burned is calculated and rounded to the nearest 10.
- The percentage is then multiplied by 10 to get the number of ml per hour of crystalloid.
- This formula is used for adults weighing 88 to 154 lb (40 to 70 kg). With patients that exceed the weight range, for each 22 lb (10 kg) in body weight over 154 lbs (70 kg), an additional 100 ml per hour is given.

Regardless of which method is used to calculate fluid requirements, this is only an estimate of fluid needs; the actual volume given must be adjusted based on the clinical response of the patient.

Pain Management

Use a multimodal analgesia strategy including both pharmacologic and nonpharmacologic interventions. Nonpharmacologic analgesia includes dry sterile dressings, covering the patient, creating a calming environment, and playing soothing music. When using pharmacologic analgesia, intravenous analgesics are preferred because intramuscular and oral analgesics have inconsistent absorption rates following severe burn. Opioid analgesics (e.g., morphine, fentanyl) are the preferred analgesic for acute burn injury. Use caution with morphine, however, because it can cause respiratory system depression. Ketamine 0.5 mg/kg can be used safely in burn patients every hour to augment pain control and decrease the risk of complications associated with use of narcotic analgesics. Use sedatives cautiously and follow local protocols for burn patient pain management.

Pain Management for Burn Patients

- Nonpharmacologic analgesia
  - Dry sterile dressings
  - Covering the patient
  - Calming environment
  - Music
- Pharmacologic analgesia
  - IV preferred
  - Opioids
    - Morphine—*caution!*
    - Fentanyl
  - Ketamine

Environmental Transport Considerations

- On-scene environmental care
  - Eliminate the cold/heat source.
  - Stop the burning process.
  - Expose and assess injuries.
  - Identify critical burns.
- Care during transport
  - Dress wounds.
  - Estimate total burn area.
  - Administer intravenous fluids.
  - Determining analgesia.
  - Prevent infection.
  - Control continuous rewarming (burns).

CASE STUDY: TRANSPORT AND ONGOING MANAGEMENT

The patient has been packaged and is ready for transport. You continuously reassess and monitor the patient, being sure to maintain normothermia. You are concerned about the patient's airway patency due to smoke inhalation. You need to provide fluid resuscitation and pain management; however, you are not able to identify any veins to establish an IV line due to both upper extremities having partial-thickness burns.

The patient is in a great deal of pain, and you provide the appropriate pain management. You also estimate the burn area size as well as burn locations to decide where you should transport the patient.

Questions:

- How will you provide fluid resuscitation?
- How will you provide pain management for this patient?
- Would you transport the patient to the nearest trauma center or a burn center?

FOR MORE INFORMATION

Refer to the "Management" section of Chapter 13: Burn Injuries in the PHTLS 10th edition main text.

CASE STUDY: WRAP-UP

Based on the location and TBSA of the burns, the patient was transported to the nearest burn center, with reassessment and monitoring performed en route. Upon arrival, the patient's burns were debrided and antimicrobial wound dressings were applied; fluid resuscitation continued for 48 hours to compensate for continued body losses. The patient was eventually discharged to a rehabilitation facility.

SUMMARY

- Exposing an injured patient is an important step in the primary survey.

- Heat loss can lead to hypothermia.

- Bariatric, geriatric, and pediatric patients require special consideration for exposure.

- Assess burns for severity and size after stopping the burning process.

- Consider the importance of pain management in patients with traumatic burn injuries.

CASE STUDY RECAP

Dispatch	
What possible injuries to the patient do you expect given the scenario?	- Burns, including inhalation injuries

Initial Impression	
What are your concerns for this patient?	- Inhalation injuries, burns, hypothermia, shock, fractures

Primary Survey	
What are the life threats with this patient?	- Burns—potential for fluid loss leading to shock, hypothermia
Is airway management indicated?	- At this point the patient is maintaining his airway; however, supplemental oxygen should be provided, because there is concern for smoke inhalation and potential for airway swelling.

What critical actions should you take?	■ Supplemental oxygen, fluid resuscitation, cutting away burned clothing, c-spine precautions, rapid transport
What is the estimated body surface area involved?	■ The patient is burned on the face, both upper extremities, and the anterior trunk. Each limb is approximately 9% of TBSA, the anterior trunk is 18%, and the face is approximately 4%. Therefore, the estimated TBSA burned is approximately 40%.

Detailed Assessment	
When should the secondary assessment be performed?	■ Secondary survey may be delayed due to the presence of life threats and associated treatment. ■ If other EMS practitioners are present, secondary and vitals may be performed simultaneously with management of the life threats.

Transport and Ongoing Management	
How will you provide fluid resuscitation?	■ Both upper extremities have partial full-thickness burns. You are not able to identify any veins to establish an IV line. ■ Neither leg is burned; however, there is an open fracture to the right ankle. ■ An IO line is started in the left tibia, and an infusion of lactated Ringer solution is started.
How will you provide pain management for this patient?	■ Fentanyl 0.1 mg/kg for pain relief and ketamine 0.5 mg/kg to augment pain control
Would you transport to the nearest trauma center or to a burn center?	■ Per the American Burn Association and the American College of Surgeons, this patient meets criteria for referral to a burn center.

STUDY QUESTIONS

1. You and your partner are responding to a call for a 2-year-old patient with a burn injury to the hand. He has a visible burn to the left hand, ending at the level above the wrist, red color, and wet in appearance. What type of burn do you suspect the patient has sustained?
   A. Superficial (first degree)
   B. Partial thickness (second degree)
   C. Full thickness (third degree)
   D. Subdermal (fourth degree)

2. The patient's caregiver is a babysitter who reports the child was crawling on the counter and placed his hand in a pot of water that was boiling on the stove. She is applying ice to the burn and the child is shivering. What is your next step?
   A. Administer analgesia for pain.
   B. Cover the patient with a blanket to stop the shivering.

   C. Start IV for fluid resuscitation.
   D. Stop the burning process and remove the ice pack.

3. After exposing the patient, no other burn injuries were found, but blisters have started to form on the hand and the child is crying from pain. How should you manage the blisters?
   A. Lance the blisters to drain the fluid and relieve the pressure.
   B. Cover the injury with a dry, loose, sterile dressing, being sure to leave the blisters intact.
   C. Use a topical antibiotic ointment and firmly wrap the burn injury.
   D. Establish an IV for fluid resuscitation.

ANSWER KEY

Question 1: B

Scald burns are the most common burns seen in the pediatric population ages 1 to 5 years. Scalds are partial-thickness burns. The dermal layer is damaged, and blisters are present or popped. It is also the most painful type of burn.

Question 2: D

A common error that results in damage to the zone of stasis is the application of ice by a bystander or prehospital care practitioner. When ice is applied to a burn, the patient will experience some reduction in pain; however, the pain relief will be at the expense of additional tissue destruction.

Question 3: B

In the prehospital setting, blisters are generally best left alone during the relatively short transport time. Blisters that have already ruptured should be covered with a clean, dry dressing.

REFERENCES AND FURTHER READING

National Association of Emergency Medical Technicians. *PHTLS: Prehospital Trauma Life Support*. 10th ed. Burlington, MA: Public Safety Group; 2023.

CHAPTER 7

Pain Management and Additional Injuries

LESSON OBJECTIVES

- Identify medications used in pain management for trauma patients.
- Explain approaches to pain management in trauma patients.
- Describe the assessment and management of patients with abdominal injuries.
- Explain the assessment and management of an obstetric patient with traumatic injuries.
- Describe the assessment and management of patients with musculoskeletal injuries.

Introduction

This lesson will include a discussion on pain management techniques, including common medications used to manage pain. Abdominal, musculoskeletal, and obstetric trauma disorders will also be reviewed.

> **QUICK TIP**
>
> Any time a pain management technique is used, EMS practitioners should continue to monitor for both therapeutic effects and adverse effects.

Pain Management

Pain is considered to be the fifth vital sign and is a complex, subjective experience. Providing adequate pain relief is one of the Golden Principles of PHTLS. EMS practitioners must rely on the patient to provide information on the type and degree of pain they are experiencing.

All patients experience pain differently because pain tolerance and thresholds vary according to the patient, hence the saying, "All pain is not the same." What might be an 8 on a scale of 1–10 to one patient could be experienced as a 6 to another. The goal for prehospital pain management in trauma patients is to use the most appropriate and effective pain management technique necessary to manage the patient's pain comfortably.

Prior to providing pain management, an EMS practitioner should identify subjective and objective patient findings to support treatment, just as with any other prehospital intervention. Keep in mind that patients have the right to pain management, and that EMS practitioners have the means to impact a patient's experience of pain and suffering.

Subjective Versus Objective

As noted, pain is primarily a subjective experience. Subjective methods for assessing pain include having the patient rate their pain from 0 to 10 (with 0 being no pain and 10 being the most pain they have ever experienced) or using the FLACC or Wong-Baker FACES pain scale for pediatric patients.

Although pain is a subjective experience, objective findings of pain include guarding, tensing on palpation, grimacing, wincing, distorted facial expressions, moaning, groaning, crying, or flushed skin.

Nonpharmacologic Pain Management

Prehospital pain management includes nonpharmacologic and pharmacologic interventions. Nonpharmacologic options include distraction, positioning, breathing techniques, and calming techniques.

Table 7-1 FLACC Pain Scale

	0 points	1 point	2 points
Face	Smiling or no particular expression	Occasional grimace or frown, withdrawn, disinterested	Frequent to constant quivering chin, clenched jaw
Legs	Normal position or relaxed	Uneasy, restless, tense	Kicking or legs drawn up
Activity	Lying quietly, normal position, moves easily	Squirming, shifting back and forth, tense	Arched, rigid, or jerking
Cry	No cry (awake or asleep)	Moans or whimpers; occasional complaint	Crying steadily, screams or sobs, frequent complaints
Consolability	Content, relaxed	Reassured by occasional touching, hugging, or being talked to; distractible	Difficult to console or comfort

Reproduced from Merkel S, Voepel-Lewis T, Shayevitz JR, & Malviya S. (1997). The FLACC: A behavioral scale for scoring postoperative pain in young children. *Pediatric Nurse*. 23(3), 293–297. Copyright © 2002, The Regents of the University of Michigan. All Rights Reserved.

Wong-Baker FACES® Pain Rating Scale

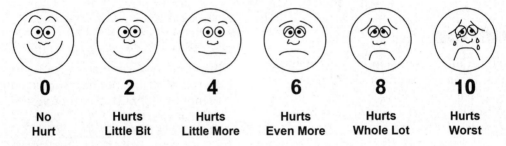

0	2	4	6	8	10
No Hurt	Hurts Little Bit	Hurts Little More	Hurts Even More	Hurts Whole Lot	Hurts Worst

Figure 7-1 Wong-Baker FACES pain scale.

© 1983 Wong-Baker FACES® Foundation. https://wongbakerfaces.org/, Used with permission. Originally published in *Whaley & Wong's Nursing Care of Infants and Children*. © Elsevier Inc.

Pediatric Pain Scales

The FLACC pain scale is recommended for patients ages 2 to 7 and assesses the **F**ace, **L**egs, **A**ctivity, **C**ry, and **C**onsolability (**Table 7-1**). The FLACC scale uses a point system to assess pain: 0 is no pain, 1–3 is mild discomfort, 4–6 is moderate pain, and 7–10 is severe pain or discomfort.

The Wong-Baker FACES pain scale features faces for children to point at that demonstrate their level of pain (**Figure 7-1**). This scale is a useful alternative for children or patients who may not be able to communicate verbally. It is available in a number of skin tones, and practitioners should have access to scales that reflect the pediatric patients in their region. The images on the FACES pain scale are intended to convey a range from "no hurt" to "hurts worst."

- Dimming the lights in the patient compartment can alleviate the stress associated with pain.
- Placing a patient in a position of comfort can help with pain relief.
- Pain or anxiety may increase a patient's ventilatory rate. Helping the patient with breathing techniques may help alleviate minor pain.
- Infants and younger children may benefit from options such as a pacifier, holding or rocking them, soft music, or repositioning.

Applying cold packs (**Figure 7-2**), splinting fractures, and applying traction splints as appropriate based on the injury are also extremely effective nonpharmacologic ways to control pain.

Pharmacologic Pain Management

It was once thought that providing pain relief would mask the patient's symptoms and impair the ability of

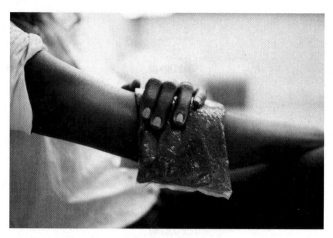

Figure 7-2 Cold pack application.
© Andrey_Popov/Shutterstock

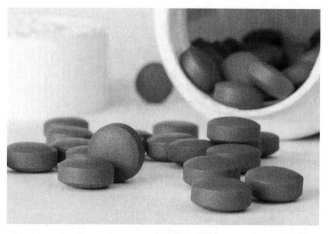

Figure 7-3 Ibuprofen is a common NSAID.
© Michelle Lee Photography/Shutterstock

the trauma team to adequately assess the patient after arrival to the hospital. Numerous studies have shown that this is not the case.

Prehospital care practitioners should consider providing analgesics to relieve pain as long as no contraindications exist. Pharmacologic treatments include opioids (e.g., fentanyl and morphine) and nonopioids (e.g., NSAIDs and ketamine). Selecting the appropriate medication for a patient is determined by multiple factors, including drug availability, drug class, mechanism of action, pharmacokinetics, pharmacodynamics, hemodynamic stability, route of administration, and of course, local protocols.

Nonopioid medications such as NSAIDs and acetaminophen should be considered as first-line treatment for mild to moderate pain. Acetaminophen can be paired with opioids to improve analgesia effects. It is commonly administered orally.

NSAIDs such as ibuprofen (**Figure 7-3**) and ketorolac can be considered. NSAIDs are beneficial for pain because they have anti-inflammatory properties and can be used in conjunction with acetaminophen for the synergistic effects. NSAIDs should be avoided in pregnant patients due to increased risk of miscarriage in early pregnancy and the premature closure of the ductus arteriosus in later stages. Ibuprofen is administered orally and provides analgesic effects within an hour. Ketorolac is administered IV and provides analgesic effects in less than 30 minutes.

Opioid medications such as fentanyl, morphine, and hydromorphone can be considered for patients experiencing moderate to severe pain and are often considered to be primary agents for managing pain. These medications should be used sparingly and should be carefully titrated to provide pain relief.

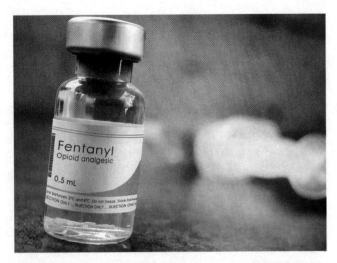

Figure 7-4 Fentanyl is often favored over morphine for pain relief based on its speed of onset, short duration of action, and minimal effect on hemodynamics.
© Sonis Photography/Shutterstock

Fentanyl

Fentanyl (**Figure 7-4**) is often a first-line agent due to speed of onset, short duration of action, and minimal effect on hemodynamics. Specific adverse effects include respiratory and circulatory depression, somnolence, constipation, weakness, and urinary retention. If fentanyl is administered too quickly, it can cause chest wall rigidity. One-time doses are not known to have an increased risk of birth defects in pregnant patients.

Consider whether the benefits outweigh the risks prior to administering this medication, and follow your local protocols. Fentanyl administered intranasally or intramuscularly has an onset time of < 10 minutes. The duration of fentanyl is short at 30 minutes to an hour.

Morphine

Morphine can be used for pain management if within local protocols; however, it has a greater risk of hypotension than fentanyl due to the profound release of histamine when administered. Specific adverse effects include respiratory and circulatory depression, bronchospasm, dizziness, urinary retention, nausea, itchiness, and constipation.

Morphine can be administered IV or IM and has a longer onset than fentanyl but also has a much longer duration of 2 to 3 hours when given IV. Morphine (0.1 mg per kg body weight) in adequate dosages may be considered for pain control in patients with traumatic burn injuries.

Ketamine

Another attractive option is a subdissociative dose (analgesic dose) of ketamine, because of its favorable

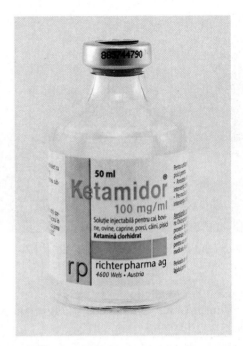

Figure 7-5 An analgesic dose of ketamine has a favorable safety profile.
© Todorean-Gabriel/Shutterstock

safety profile that maintains hemodynamic stability and respiratory drive when appropriately administered. Ketamine is an N-methyl-d-aspartate (NMDA) receptor antagonist that has gained popularity in the management of pain. Its benefits over opioids include bronchodilation and stimulation of the sympathetic nervous system and cardiovascular system.

Ketamine can be administered intravenously or intranasally (**Figure 7-5**). Dosing needs will vary by patient according to the desired effect, the patient's age, and underlying conditions. Dosing adjustments will be required if used in combination with other medications, such as morphine or fentanyl.

Adverse effects include hypertension and tachycardia. In rare cases, ketamine has been shown to cause laryngospasm and an increase in intraocular pressure.

Caution should be used when administering ketamine to patients who have ingested substances such as cocaine, alcohol, amphetamines, ecstasy, opiates, and synthetic cathinone because they have an increased likelihood of requiring intubation after ketamine administration.

Abdominal Trauma

The abdomen is the third most commonly injured body region in trauma. EMS practitioners should maintain an understanding of the major organs in the abdomen to identify internal injuries. There is limited protection to the abdominal organs, more specifically to the lateral and anterior positions.

Dividing the organs into hollow, solid, and vascular groups can help explain symptoms of injuries to these organs. Solid organs and blood vessels will bleed into the abdominal cavity when injured, potentially leading to hemorrhagic shock. Hollow organs will primarily spill their contents into the peritoneal cavity and retroperitoneal space, resulting in peritonitis and sepsis.

A brief anatomy review of the organs in the peritoneal and retroperitoneal space can help identify which organs may be impacted in trauma (**Figure 7-6**):

- Peritoneal cavity
  - Solid
    - Liver: RUQ and LUQ
    - Spleen: LUQ
  - Hollow
    - Stomach: RUQ and LUQ
    - Gallbladder: RUQ
    - Large intestine (transverse and sigmoid colon): RUQ, LUQ, and LLQ
    - Small intestine (jejunum and ileum): RUQ, LUQ, LLQ, and RLQ
    - Female reproductive organs: RLQ and LLQ

- Retroperitoneal space
  - Solid
    - Kidneys: RUQ and LUQ
    - Pancreas: RUQ and LUQ
  - Vascular
    - Inferior vena cava: RUQ and LUQ
    - Abdominal aorta: RUQ and LUQ
    - Iliac arteries and veins: RLQ and LLQ
  - Hollow
    - Large intestine (ascending and descending colon): RLQ and LLQ
    - Small intestine (duodenum): RUQ
    - Rectum: RLQ and LLQ
    - Ureters: RLQ and LLQ

Penetrating Trauma

Most penetrating trauma results from stab and gunshot wounds. High-velocity injuries, such as those created by high-powered rifles and assault weapons, tend to create more serious injuries because of the larger temporary cavities created as the projectile moves through the peritoneal cavity. Projectiles may strike bones (ribs, spine, or pelvis), resulting in fragments that may perforate internal organs. Stab wounds are less likely to penetrate the peritoneal cavity than projectiles fired from a handgun, rifle, or shotgun. Stab wounds are more likely to

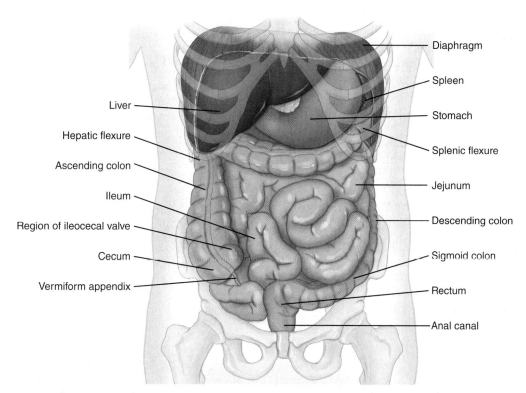

Figure 7-6 Organs in the peritoneal cavity include solid organs (spleen and liver), hollow organs of the gastrointestinal tract (stomach, small intestine, and colon), and reproductive organs.

damage—in order of frequency—the liver, small bowel, and diaphragm, whereas gunshot wounds are more likely to damage the small bowel, colon, and liver.

Blast Injuries

A primary blast injury to the abdomen is most likely to affect the hollow organs—likely a bowel wall injury—and may present with delayed symptoms such as bowel wall necrosis or perforation. Secondary blast injuries may occur due to debris penetrating the abdomen. Tertiary blast injuries are similar to blunt trauma, as when a person is thrown against an object, and may result in splenic, renal, or hepatic lacerations.

Blunt Trauma

Blunt trauma results from compression or shear forces and can be challenging to identify. Compression injuries are caused by the abdominal organs being crushed between solid objects. Increased intra-abdominal pressure can rupture the diaphragm, causing abdominal organs to move upward into the thoracic cavity, affecting respiratory and cardiac activity. Tearing forces exerted against their supporting ligaments can rupture blood vessels and/or solid organs in the abdomen from shear forces.

Location of impact and objects that the patient could have encountered during a traumatic event should be considered when assessing a patient suspected of sustaining blunt trauma. For instance, a driver-side impact in a motor vehicle collision should increase suspicion for a splenic injury versus a possible liver injury that would be suspected from a passenger-side impact. Deceleration and compression injuries should be suspected in a head-on collision.

Physical examination is a critical piece of assessment to identify and manage abdominal trauma when used in conjunction with the mechanism of injury and bystander and patient information provided on scene. The abdomen should be fully exposed and examined for any evidence of trauma, because there are limited diagnostic capabilities available in the prehospital setting.

Primary Survey

Most severe abdominal injuries present as abnormalities identified in the primary survey, primarily in the evaluation of breathing and circulation. Unless there are associated injuries, patients with abdominal trauma generally present with a patent airway. The alterations found in the breathing, circulation, and disability assessments generally correspond to the degree of shock present; that is, increased respiratory rate, tachycardia, hypotension, and pale, cool skin can all be clinical indicators of abdominal trauma (**Figure 7-7**).

Secondary Survey

Inspection during the secondary survey includes looking for any distension and soft tissue injuries such as contusions, abrasions, penetrating wounds, obvious bleeding, and uncommon findings such as evisceration, impaled objects, or tire marks.

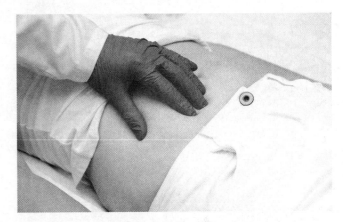

Figure 7-7 Fully expose the abdomen to examine for evidence of trauma.
© HENADZI KILENT/Shutterstock

The "seat belt sign" (ecchymosis or abrasion across the abdomen resulting from compression of the abdominal wall against a shoulder harness or lap belt) indicates that significant force was applied to the abdomen as a result of sudden deceleration and increases the likelihood of intra-abdominal injury eightfold (**Figure 7-8**). A pediatric patient presenting with the seat belt sign is much more likely to have an intra-abdominal injury than an adult.

Grey-Turner sign (ecchymosis involving the flanks) and Cullen sign (ecchymosis around the umbilicus) indicate retroperitoneal bleeding; however, these signs will most often be delayed and may not be seen in the initial few hours following an injury.

Palpation is used to identify abdominal tenderness either globally or to a specific area/region (**Figure 7-9**). EMS practitioners should begin palpating in the quadrant where the patient does not have pain and then in each quadrant thereafter.

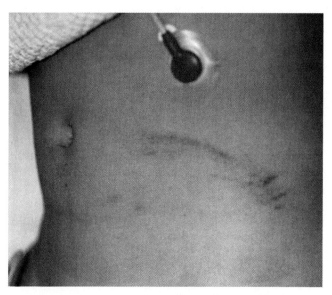

Figure 7-8 An abdominal "seat belt sign" resulting from the patient decelerating against a lap belt.
Courtesy of Peter T. Pons, MD, FACEP.

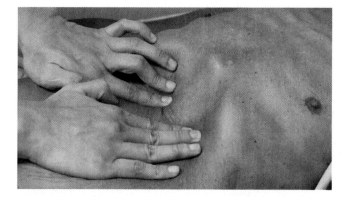

Figure 7-9 Abdominal palpation.
© Casa nayafana/Shutterstock

While palpating, EMS practitioners should identify any voluntary or involuntary guarding.

- Involuntary guarding is indicated with rigidity or spasm of the abdominal wall muscles due to peritonitis.
- Voluntary guarding is noted when the patient tenses up the abdominal muscles to protect from pain as a result of palpation.

Avoid deep or aggressive palpation to prevent causing more pain and to avoid aggravating bleeding or other injuries. A palpated exam in patients with an altered mental status may be unreliable, because they may be unable to accurately report pain or tenderness.

Palpating the pelvis is not necessary in the prehospital setting, but if done should only be performed once due to the potential for disruption of any clots that have formed at the site of a fracture, potentially exacerbating internal hemorrhage. The procedure for pelvic palpation is a two-step process and should be performed using gentle pressure to identify any tenderness or instability:

1. Pressing inward on the iliac crests
2. Pressing posteriorly on the pubic symphysis

Management of Abdominal Injuries

A critical aspect of managing abdominal trauma is identifying the presence of the injury and rapidly transporting the patient to the most appropriate facility.

Abdominal trauma with hypotension or peritoneal signs, evisceration, or an impaled object indicates the need for surgical intervention, and these patients should be transported to a trauma facility with immediate surgical capabilities. Hemodynamically unstable patients who have sustained blunt trauma and have a suspected pelvic injury should be managed with a commercial pelvic binder (or sheet) to stabilize and secure the pelvis to reduce the risk of major hemorrhage during transport.

EMS practitioners must use caution when providing fluid resuscitation en route. A delicate balance is necessary to maintain a blood pressure that allows for perfusion to the vital organs without restoring blood pressure to normal or elevated ranges, which could "pop a clot," leading to increased bleeding in the abdomen and pelvis. In the absence of traumatic brain injury (TBI), the target systolic blood pressure is 80 to 90 mm Hg (mean arterial pressure of 60 to 65 mm Hg). For patients with suspected intra-abdominal bleeding and a TBI, the systolic blood pressure is maintained at a minimum of 110 mm Hg.

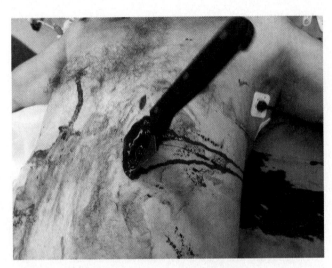

Figure 7-10 Removal of an impaled object from the abdomen is contraindicated in the prehospital environment.
Courtesy of Lance Stuke, MD, MPH.

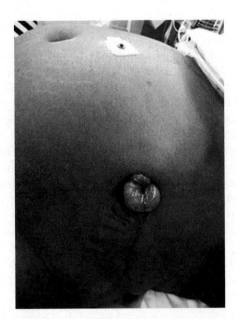

Figure 7-11 Bowel eviscerated through a wound in the abdominal wall.
Courtesy of Lance Stuke, MD, MPH.

Special Considerations in Abdominal Injuries

Impaled Objects

The removal of an impaled object is contraindicated in the prehospital setting (**Figure 7-10**), because it could be actively controlling bleeding (tamponade effect). To prevent movement in the field and during transport, the impaled object should be mechanically or manually stabilized. If the object requires cutting to free the patient and initiate transport, the EMS practitioner should apply direct pressure manually around the object and monitor the patient closely for additional bleeding internally or externally.

Evisceration

In the presence of evisceration, do not attempt to replace the protruding tissue back into the abdominal cavity (**Figure 7-11**). The viscera should be left as found and covered with clean or sterile dressing that has been moistened with saline to prevent cellular death. The dressings should be monitored during transport and remoistened as needed to prevent them from drying out. To maintain patient normothermia, wet dressings can be covered with a large dry or occlusive dressing.

Efforts should be made to keep the patient calm, because any increase in abdominal pressure resulting from screaming, crying, or coughing could force more organs out of the abdomen.

Obstetric Trauma

Motor vehicles account for half of all traumatic injuries during pregnancy and 82% of trauma related to fetal death. The improper use of seat belts is the main reason for many of these accidents. Pelvic fracture is the most common maternal injury that leads to fetal death.

Many anatomic and physiologic changes occur throughout pregnancy that can alter the pattern of injuries and the body's normal response to trauma. EMS practitioners could be managing two or more patients and must be aware of the changes that occur throughout pregnancy.

The following are relevant anatomic and physiologic changes:

- Circulatory changes
  - Red blood cell volume could increase by 30% at term gestation.
  - 50% increase of cardiac output by 8 weeks.
  - 30% increase in stroke volume by the third trimester.
  - 80% increase in plasma volume to the kidneys during the second trimester.
  - Blood volume to the liver and brain is *not* increased during pregnancy.
- Respiratory changes
  - Functional residual capacity (FRC) can decrease anywhere from 10% to 25% during pregnancy.
  - Tidal volume increases up to 45%.
  - Minute ventilation will also increase.

- Renal changes
  - Due to increased cardiac output, the kidneys increase in size by about 30%.
  - The glomerular filtration rate (GFR) increases 50% more than normal due to the increase in renal blood flow.
- Gastrointestinal changes
  - A reduction in esophageal sphincter tone leads to a higher risk of reflux of gastric contents due to the stomach rotating and becoming displaced during pregnancy.
  - Decrease in peristalsis increases the risk for vomiting and aspiration.

- Endocrine changes
  - Increase in progesterone allows for systemic vasodilation and decrease in blood pressure.
  - Thyroid hormone increases to about 50% more than normal.
  - Endorphins and enkephalin increase to allow for a higher pain threshold.
  - Free cortisol levels increase to 2.5 times higher.
- Uterus
  - A gravid uterus and placenta are extremely vascular, which could cause excessive hemorrhage with any associated injuries.

Physical Examination

Inspection, Palpation, and Auscultation

By the 20th week of gestation, the top of the uterus (fundus) is observed to be at the umbilicus; by 38 weeks it approaches the xiphoid process (**Figure 7-12**), making the uterus and its contents more susceptible to blunt and penetrating injury. Injuries to the uterus can include rupture, abruptio placentae, penetration, and premature rupture of the membranes.

Trauma is the most common cause of abruptio placentae (even minor motor vehicle collisions and/or falls). You should have a high degree of suspicion with any form of trauma, especially in the last trimester of pregnancy. A firm, hard, and tender uterus is suggestive of abruptio placentae, with vaginal bleeding visible in 70% of cases. Hemorrhage may be concealed within the uterus or peritoneal cavity, leaving no external visible sign present on inspection (**Figure 7-13**).

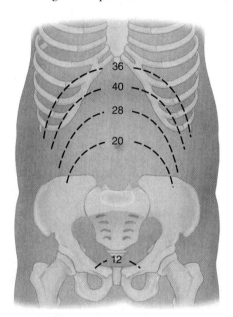

Figure 7-12 Fundal height. As pregnancy progresses, the uterus becomes more susceptible to injury.

© National Association of Emergency Medical Technicians (NAEMT)

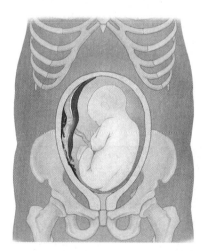
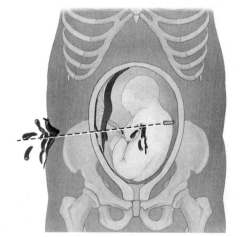
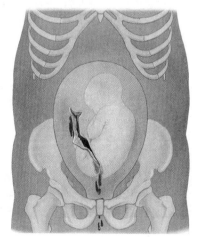

A   **B**   **C**

Figure 7-13 Diagram of uterine trauma. **A.** Abruptio placentae. **B.** Gunshot to the uterus. **C.** Ruptured uterus.

© National Association of Emergency Medical Technicians (NAEMT)

Due to the increase in blood volume and cardiac output, a pregnant patient could lose 1,200 to 1,500 ml of blood before exhibiting signs and symptoms of hypovolemia. Hypovolemic shock may induce premature labor in patients in the third trimester. Look for subtle changes such as skin color and alterations in mental status when assessing for signs of significant bleeding. During a traumatic event, the body will shunt blood away from the fetus to provide for the vital organs. Avoid wasting valuable time trying to identify the absence or presence of fetal heart tones, because this would not change your management of the patient and would delay care.

Ask the patient whether contractions are occurring or if there has been a decrease in fetal movement. Contractions could indicate premature labor, and decreased fetal movement could be a sign that the fetus is in distress.

Management of Obstetric Injuries

Some women may have significant hypotension when supine. This supine hypotension of pregnancy typically occurs in the third trimester and is caused by the compression of the inferior vena cava by the enlarged uterus.

Three maneuvers can be used to relieve supine hypotension (**Figure 7-14**):

- Place the patient on her left side (lateral decubitus).
- Manual left uterine displacement.
- Elevate right leg (to displace uterus to the left).

Manage the patient's life threats found during the primary survey.

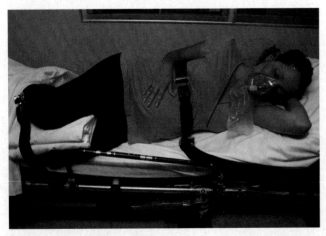

Figure 7-14 Tipping a pregnant woman onto her left side helps displace the uterus from the inferior vena cava and improves blood return to the heart, thus restoring blood pressure.

© Jones & Bartlett Learning. Courtesy of MIEMSS.

QUICK TIP

Keep in mind that focusing on the obstetric patient is the best management for the fetus, because generally the patient must survive in order for the fetus to survive.

Shock management is the same for obstetric patients as for nonpregnant patients; however, restoring the blood pressure to a normal systolic and mean pressure will promote greater fetal perfusion, despite the risk of promoting additional internal hemorrhage in the patient. Pregnant trauma patients should be transported to the closest appropriate facility, ideally a trauma center with surgical and obstetric capabilities.

Resuscitative cesarean delivery is indicated in patients in traumatic arrest who are 24 weeks or greater and can be performed by ED physicians. At 24 weeks the fetus is viable.

When performing basic and advanced life support (e.g., CPR) on an obstetric patient, ensure that left uterine displacement is performed to facilitate effective perfusion. The goal to deliver is within 5 minutes postarrest due to the decline in neurologic recovery of the newborn. Calling an OB alert to the receiving facility in cases of traumatic arrest will prepare the hospital staff to provide essential care to the OB patient.

CASE STUDY: DISPATCH

You and your partner work for a suburban EMS agency. You are dispatched to a two-car motor vehicle collision (MVC) during morning rush hour. It is 0800 on a cool morning with an outside temperature of 50°F (10°C). Patient is a 24-year-old female at 36 weeks' gestation, approximately 190 lb (86 kg). There is a Level II trauma center with labor and delivery services 8 minutes away by ground.

Question:

- What are your questions and concerns based on the dispatch information?

CASE STUDY: INITIAL IMPRESSION

You arrive at the scene to find that two vehicles have pulled over to a parking lot off the road. Law enforcement is on scene. The patient was a front-seat passenger in a small sedan that rear-ended a stopped SUV at a speed of approximately 30 mph (48 kph). There is exterior front-end damage to the sedan. The air bags in the sedan deployed, and the passenger was wearing a seat belt. Fire personnel arrive within minutes after you. All others involved in the MVC are not injured.

Questions:

- What are your concerns for this patient?
- What potential injuries do you suspect?

Musculoskeletal Trauma

The skeletal system is divided into two primary divisions: the axial and appendicular systems (**Figure 7-15**). The axial system includes the skull, spine, sternum, and ribs. The appendicular system includes the bones of all extremities, the shoulder girdle, and the pelvis.

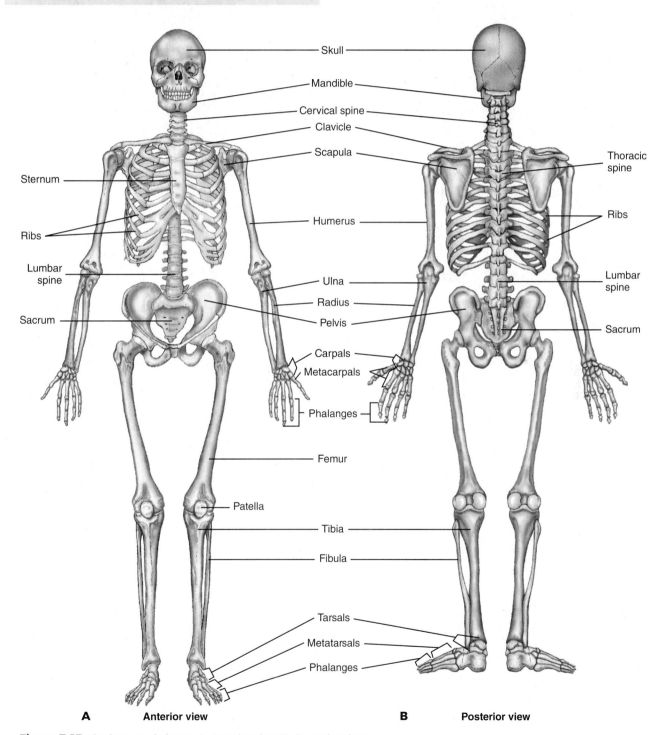

A   **Anterior view**   **B**   **Posterior view**

Figure 7-15 The human skeleton. **A.** Anterior view. **B.** Posterior view.

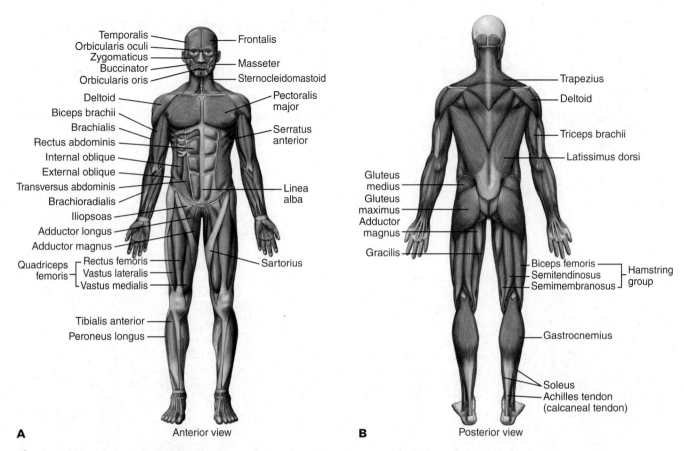

Figure 7-16 Major muscles of the human body. **A.** Anterior view. **B.** Posterior view.

© National Association of Emergency Medical Technicians (NAEMT)

The muscular system is divided into voluntary and involuntary muscles (**Figure 7-16**). Voluntary muscles are also known as skeletal muscles because they move the skeletal system. Involuntary muscles do not move or contract with conscious control. Also within the musculoskeletal system are tendons and ligaments. Tendons are inelastic fibrous tissues that connect a muscle to a bone. Ligaments are bands of fibrous tissue connecting bone to bone with the purpose of keeping joints together.

Assessment

There are three types of musculoskeletal trauma:

- Life-threatening injuries
- Non–life-threatening injuries associated with multisystem life-threatening trauma
- Isolated non–life-threatening injuries

Primary Survey

When performing the primary survey, avoid the pitfall of "tunnel vision" focused on angulated fractures or partial amputations (dramatic injuries; **Figure 7-17**) rather than first assessing and managing life-threatening conditions. Exsanguinating hemorrhage is often due to a musculoskeletal injury and should be treated with compression or tourniquet placement.

Secondary Survey

The examination and management of extremities occurs during the secondary survey. Clothing that was not removed during the primary survey to address life-threatening injuries should be removed during the secondary survey for an effective examination to occur. The secondary survey includes identifying any pain, weakness, or abnormal sensations in the extremities.

Assessment of the extremities should include examining for dislocations or fractures by palpating bones and joints for any tenderness or crepitus. Common joint dislocation deformities may occur at the shoulder, elbow, hip, knee, and ankle.

Look for swelling, lacerations, abrasions, skin color, and hematomas to determine if soft tissue injuries are present. Document the size, color, and location of wounds. Perfusion can be assessed by evaluating the distal pulses of all extremities for pulse presence, regularity, and strength. Capillary refill in the fingers or toes should also be assessed.

Examine for motor and sensory functions of all extremities as part of your neurologic assessment. Motor function can initially be evaluated by asking the patient about any areas of weakness. The patient's grip strength is tested by asking them to squeeze the examiner's finger. The lower extremities are evaluated by the patient's ability to wiggle their toes and the push–pull of their feet against the examiner's hands.

Sensory function is examined by asking the patient if there are any deficits or changes in sensation. Sensation should be tested at the distal end of each extremity.

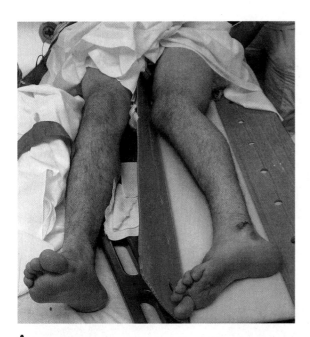

A

B

Figure 7-17 A. Closed fracture of the femur. Note the internal rotation and shortening of the left leg. **B.** Open fracture of the tibia.

CASE STUDY: PRIMARY SURVEY

- **X**—No major external hemorrhage noted
- **A**—Patent
- **B**—24, shallow
- **C**—116, strong radial pulses; skin pale, warm, and dry
- **D**—GCS 15 (E4, V5, M6); PERRL; pain is 8/10
- **E**—Notable bruising to abdomen, abdominal rigidity noted, powder burns to face from airbag deployment

Questions:

- What are the potential life threats given the mechanism of injury and primary survey results?
- How many patients do you have?

Management of Musculoskeletal Injuries

Fractures

Fractures are classified as open (bone is functionally or grossly exposed) or closed (integrity of skin remains intact; **Figure 7-18**).

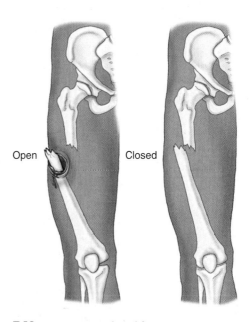

Open   Closed

Figure 7-18 Open versus closed fracture.

After controlling hemorrhage and treating for shock, open wounds or exposed bone ends should be gently rinsed with saline or sterile water to remove contamination and covered with a saline- or water-moistened sterile dressing. If possible, return the limb to its normal anatomic alignment. Realigning a deformed extremity prior to splinting can help with pain control, make splinting easier, stabilize the fracture, and improve perfusion. No more than two attempts at alignment should be performed. If unsuccessful, the extremity should be splinted "as is." Consider analgesia such as fentanyl when realigning a deformed extremity prior to splinting.

The primary objective of splinting a deformity is to limit movement of the fractured body part. To effectively immobilize any long bone in an extremity, the entire limb should be immobilized. To do this, the injured site should be supported manually while the joint and bone above (proximal to) and the joint and bone below (distal to) the injury site are immobilized. Numerous types of splints are available (**Figure 7-19**), and most can be used with both open and closed fractures. Document any bone ends that retract into the wound and report to ED staff.

Keep in mind these four critical points to applying a splint:

1. Use padded splints or add padding to prevent movement, increase patient comfort, and prevent pressure sores.
2. Remove jewelry that could potentially inhibit circulation with continued swelling.
3. Assess neurovascular function before and after applying a splint. Continue to monitor throughout care.
4. Ice or cold packs could be used to decrease pain and swelling by placing them on the splinted extremity near the suspected fracture site.

Pulseless Extremities

The EMS practitioner should make one attempt to realign the limb to normal anatomic appearance in a patient who presents with a deformed limb without a pulse (**Figure 7-20A**). Pain management should be considered prior to attempting limb realignment. Pulses should then be rechecked to see if blood flow has been restored to the limb. The limb should then be splinted in place (**Figure 7-20B**).

> ### QUICK TIP
>
> A pulseless extremity is a limb-threatening injury, and the patient should be transported to a facility with immediate surgical capabilities.

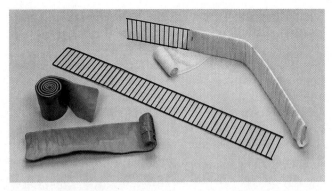

A

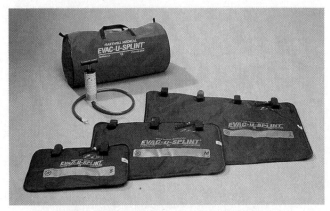

B

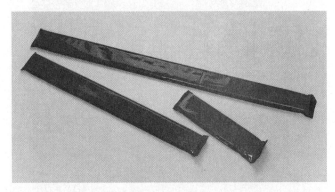

C

Figure 7-19 A. Formable splint. **B.** Vacuum splint. **C.** Board splint.

A and **C.** © National Association of Emergency Medical Technicians (NAEMT); **B.** Courtesy of Hartwell Medical.

Pelvic Fracture

Pelvic fractures can range from minor to life-threatening. Patients with pelvic fractures frequently have associated injuries, including traumatic brain injuries, long-bone fractures, thoracic injuries, urethral disruption in men, splenic trauma, and liver and kidney trauma.

A pelvic binder (or sheet, if a commercial binder is not available) should be applied when a significant mechanism of injury and concern for pelvic ring injury are present. The pelvic binder is designed to reduce

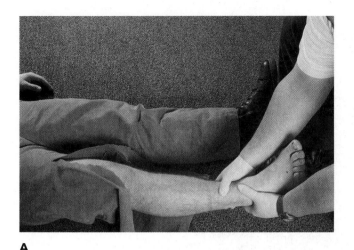

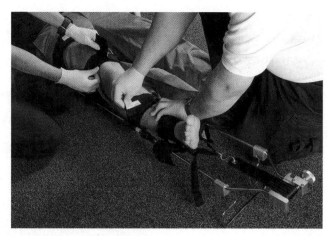

A   **B**

Figure 7-20 A. Realignment of the limb. **B.** Splinting the limb in place.
© Jones & Bartlett Learning. Photographed by Darren Stahlman.

blood loss from pelvic fractures and not for fracture stabilization. Pelvic binders are commonly placed inappropriately (too superiorly), leading to additional complications. EMS practitioners should ensure the pelvic binder is centered over the greater trochanters and not the pelvic brim. Confirming the proper location allows for the transfer of compression from the binder to the pelvis regardless of body habitus. The result of proper placement is a reduction of pelvic volume, stabilization of the pelvis, and, ideally, a decrease in ongoing bleeding.

Femur Fracture

Like pelvic injuries, femur fractures can be life threatening due to the large amount of associated hemorrhage into each thigh. A traction splint should be applied to patients suspected to have a non–life-threatening mid-shaft femur fracture. The application of traction, both manually and by use of a mechanical device, can help decrease internal bleeding as well as decrease the patient's pain.

Contraindications on the use of traction splints include:

- Avulsion or amputation of the ipsilateral ankle or foot
- Suspected fractures of the adjacent knee

Dislocations

A dislocation is a separation of two bones at the joint, resulting from significant disruption to the ligaments that normally provide supporting structure and stability at a joint. A dislocation, similar to a fracture, produces an area of instability that the prehospital care practitioner needs to secure.

A dislocation can be difficult to distinguish clinically from a fracture without radiographic evaluation and may be associated with fractures as well (fracture-dislocation). Deformity of a joint provides a clue to the type and direction of dislocation. A suspected dislocation is typically splinted in the position it was found; however, manipulation of the joint can be performed in the presence of an absent or weak pulse to improve perfusion.

When faced with a brief transport time to the hospital, however, the better decision is to initiate transport rather than attempt manipulation. This manipulation will cause the patient great pain, so the patient should be prepared before moving the extremity. A splint should be used to immobilize most dislocations, whereas a sling is used for shoulder injuries. Documentation of how the injury was sustained and found and of the presence of pulse, movement, sensation, and color before and after splinting is important. During transport, ice or cold packs can be used to decrease pain and swelling. Analgesia can be provided as necessary to reduce pain.

Manipulation of a dislocation injury should only be performed if allowed under local protocols and if done by properly trained practitioners; it also needs to be fully documented.

Compartment Syndrome

Compartment syndrome is caused by decreased blood supply to an extremity due to increased pressure within the limb. The pressure may increase to the point that arterial flow and nerve function are compromised.

The two main causes are from hemorrhage within a compartment from a fracture or vascular injury and

CASE STUDY: DETAILED ASSESSMENT

Vital Signs:

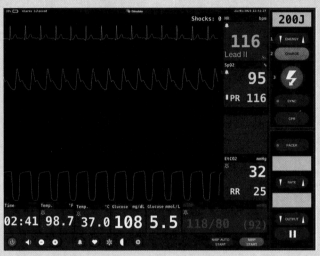

© National Association of Emergency Medical Technicians (NAEMT)

Secondary Assessment:

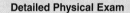

Detailed Physical Exam

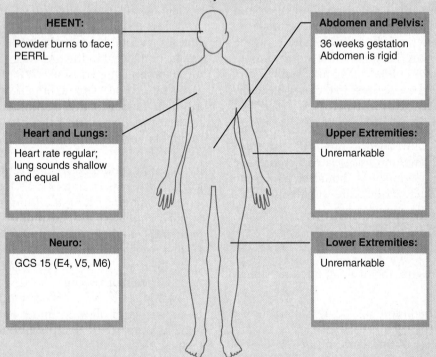

HEENT:

Powder burns to face; PERRL

Heart and Lungs:

Heart rate regular; lung sounds shallow and equal

Neuro:

GCS 15 (E4, V5, M6)

Abdomen and Pelvis:

36 weeks gestation
Abdomen is rigid

Upper Extremities:

Unremarkable

Lower Extremities:

Unremarkable

© National Association of Emergency Medical Technicians (NAEMT)

Questions:

- What are your ongoing concerns for the patient?
- What critical actions should you perform?

third space edema that is formed after ischemic muscle tissue is reperfused after a period of diminished or absent blood flow.

Signs of a patient developing compartment syndrome are:

- Pain above the baseline pain appropriate to the trauma and not relieved by pain management measures.
- Altered or reduced sensation of the involved extremity.
- Absent pulse, pale skin, and paralysis in the injured extremity are late findings.

Compartment syndrome management requires surgical intervention to decompress the affected muscle tissue. EMS practitioners should ensure any splinting or compression dressings applied are not tight, assess for distal pulses, and avoid elevating the extremity. Patients may develop compartment syndrome during long transport times, and therefore, should be monitored continuously en route to the ED.

Mangled Extremities

A "mangled extremity" is a complex injury (**Figure 7-21**). Common mechanisms of injury producing mangled extremities include high-energy transfers such as a motorcycle crash, ejection from a motor vehicle, and a pedestrian being struck by an automobile.

Most mangled extremities involve severe open fractures where amputation of the limb may be necessary. However, some limbs can be salvaged and should be managed accordingly. The focus for management of a mangled extremity should be on hemorrhage control, and a tourniquet may be required. The injury should be splinted as time allows and the patient transported to the most appropriate facility with surgical capabilities (usually a high-volume Level I trauma center).

Amputations

All amputations may be accompanied by significant bleeding, but this is more common with partial amputations. When vessels are completely transected (complete amputation; **Figure 7-22**), they retract and constrict, and blood clots may form, decreasing or stopping hemorrhage; however, when a vessel is only partially transected (partial amputation), the two ends cannot retract, and blood continues to pour out of the wound.

It is important to locate the missing extremity for possible reattachment. This is especially true for the upper extremity and thumb. Lower extremity amputations are generally not reattached in the setting of traumatic amputations because lower extremity prostheses are effective and the success of replantation in the lower extremity is poor. However, do not delay transport to search for the missing extremity. Law enforcement officials or other first responders could remain at the scene to find the amputated part and transport it to the facility that is receiving the patient.

As with any traumatic injury, focus first on hemorrhage control, airway, and breathing. Amputations can be very painful, so prepare to offer analgesia to the patient.

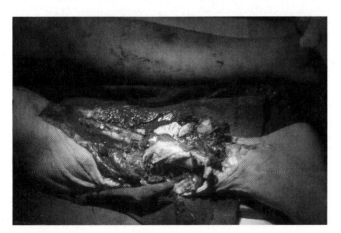

Figure 7-21 Mangled extremity resulting from a crushing injury between two vehicles. The patient has fractures and extensive soft-tissue injury.
Courtesy of Peter T. Pons, MD, FACEP.

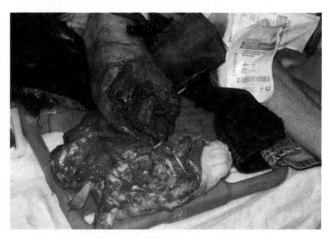

Figure 7-22 Complete amputation of the right leg after it became entangled in machinery.
Courtesy of Peter T. Pons, MD, FACEP.

Managing an amputated extremity includes:

- Gently rinse the amputated part with lactated Ringer solution.
- Wrap the part in sterile gauze moistened with lactated Ringer, place it in a container or plastic bag, and label it.
- Place the bag or container in an outer container with crushed ice to keep cool and reduce the metabolic rate, thus providing critical time.
- Avoid freezing the part—do not place it directly on ice or add another coolant such as dry ice.
- Transport the part along with the patient to the closest appropriate facility with surgical and replantation capabilities.

CASE STUDY: TRANSPORT AND ONGOING MANAGEMENT

The patient is immediately packaged and ready for transport. An IV is established. Vitals are reassessed throughout transport.

Questions:
- How would you package the patient for transport?
- What is your transport destination?
- What interventions will you perform en route?

Crush Syndrome

An extremity crushed during a traumatic event can cause rhabdomyolysis, which is associated with muscle death and the release of myoglobin. Traumatic muscle injury causes release of both myoglobin and potassium; when the crushing force is released and perfusion to the limb resumes, the blood that was trapped in the extremity, which contains higher levels of myoglobin and potassium, is washed out of the injured limb and into the rest of the body.

EMS practitioners should maintain awareness for the development of crush syndrome in patients who have experienced prolonged entrapment, traumatic injury to muscle mass, and compromised circulation to the injured area.

Early and aggressive fluid resuscitation is critical to improved patient outcomes. Therefore, resuscitation should begin prior to extrication. A poorly resuscitated patient may go into cardiac arrest during extrication because of the sudden release of metabolic acid and potassium into the bloodstream when the compression on the extremity is released. Fluid resuscitation should proceed with normal saline at a rate of 1,500 ml/hr to ensure adequate renal output of 150 to 200 ml/hr. Avoid lactated Ringer until urine output is adequate, because the solution contains potassium. Adding 50 mEq of sodium bicarbonate and 10 g of mannitol to each liter of fluid may decrease the incidence of renal failure. Once extricated, normal saline can be reduced to 500 ml/hr, alternating with D_5W, with one ampule of sodium bicarbonate per liter.

Once blood pressure is stabilized, focus is turned toward prophylactic management of hyperkalemia and the toxic effects of serum myoglobin. Hyperkalemia in the field can be recognized by the development of peaked T waves on the cardiac monitor. Treatment of the increased potassium follows standard protocols for hyperkalemia, including IV sodium bicarbonate administration, inhaled beta-agonists (albuterol), administration of dextrose and insulin (if available), and, if life-threatening cardiac dysrhythmias occur, IV calcium chloride.

CASE STUDY: WRAP-UP

Patient was transported to the nearby Level II trauma center with labor and delivery services. Fluid resuscitation was provided en route.

Uterine rupture was confirmed, an emergency cesarian delivery was performed, and the newborn was successfully delivered. Both mother and baby recovered completely.

Question:
- What is the goal of fluid resuscitation in pregnant patients?

SUMMARY

- Most patients who experience a traumatic injury are in pain and require some type of pain management technique, which could be nonpharmacologic or pharmacologic. Selecting the most appropriate method to relieve pain is necessary to achieve the best patient outcome. Effective examination and communication will ensure the best technique is used.

- EMS practitioners often have limited tools to complete a thorough abdominal assessment. Thus, patients with a suspected abdominal injury should be properly managed with expedited transport to the closest appropriate facility.

- Pregnant patients present with unique challenges that require quick and effective management to increase positive patient outcomes. Understanding the anatomic and physiologic changes to women during pregnancy is an important part of assessment and management of pregnant patients who have sustained traumatic injuries.

- Be attentive to early signs of shock in pregnant patients.

- Musculoskeletal injuries are rarely considered to be an immediate life threat; however, a thorough examination should identify when an injury produces significant external or internal bleeding, identifying a life-threatening disorder.

- Avoid tunnel vision of distracting injuries; keep focused on the patient as a whole and treat life threats.

CASE STUDY RECAP

Dispatch

What are your questions and concerns based on the dispatch information?	■ Is the scene safe? ■ How fast were the vehicles going? ■ What injuries did the patient sustain? ■ Well-being of the fetus

Initial Impression

What are your concerns for this patient?	■ Concerns include whether the patient is going into labor and the criticality of her injuries.
What potential injuries do you suspect?	■ Uterine rupture or other obstetric trauma, possible burns from airbag deployment.

Primary Survey

What are the potential life threats given the mechanism of injury and primary survey results?	■ Uterine rupture, hypovolemic shock
How many patients do you have?	■ Technically two, because the fetus is past the age of viability

Detailed Assessment

What are your ongoing concerns for the patient?	■ Because the uterus is highly vascular, there could be uterine rupture with no external bleeding visible. ■ Blood loss could lead to hypovolemic shock.
What critical actions should you perform?	■ Extrication from vehicle, rapid transport, fluid resuscitation

Transport and Ongoing Management

How would you package the patient for transport?	■ Patient was placed in left lateral recumbent position to mitigate risk of supine hypotension.
What is your transport destination?	■ Nearest trauma center with obstetric capabilities
What interventions will you perform en route?	■ Establish IV access and begin fluid resuscitation, provide supplemental oxygen, call OB alert to receiving facility.

Wrap-Up

| What is the goal of fluid resuscitation in pregnant patients? | ■ The primary goal of fluid resuscitation in a pregnant patient is to provide judicious IV fluid administration in an attempt to restore normal systolic and mean blood pressures. Doing so will likely result in better fetal perfusion, despite the risk of promoting additional internal hemorrhage in the woman. |

STUDY QUESTIONS

1. Your patient is experiencing severe pain after sustaining a femur fracture in a motorcycle crash. You have a 20-minute transport to the nearest trauma center. There are no other injuries noted on your primary and secondary assessments. Which of the following medications would be the best pain management choice?
   A. NSAIDs
   B. Acetaminophen
   C. Fentanyl
   D. Morphine

2. You are responding to a call to an MVC involving one patient. When you perform your primary survey, you find a patent airway, but abnormalities with breathing and circulation. You suspect hypovolemic shock, but cannot determine the source. What does this finding most likely indicate?
   A. Hemothorax
   B. Intra-abdominal bleed
   C. Blunt cardiac injury
   D. Diaphragmatic rupture

3. You are transporting a 37-year-old male patient with a suspected intra-abdominal bleed. His blood pressure is 70/50 mm Hg (MAP 57), and his skin is pale and diaphoretic. How will you manage fluid resuscitation for this patient?
   A. Aggressively administer IV fluids to compensate for internal blood loss.
   B. Do not administer IV fluids to patients with intra-abdominal bleeding.
   C. Obtain the patient's medical records and resuscitate to his normal blood pressure reading.
   D. Carefully administer IV fluids to raise the patient's systolic blood pressure to between 80 and 90 mm Hg.

ANSWER KEY

Question 1: C
Fentanyl is often a first-line agent due to speed of onset, short duration of action, and minimal effect on hemodynamics. Fentanyl can be administered IN, IM, IO, or IV. The IV route provides effects instantly whereas the IN and IM route have an onset of < 10 minutes. The duration of fentanyl is short at 30 minutes to an hour. This will provide enough time to ease pain during transport and let the trauma center decide pain management upon arrival.

Question 2: B
The most reliable indicator of an intra-abdominal bleed is the presence of hypovolemic shock from an unexplained source.

Question 3: D
Abdominal trauma represents one of the key situations in which a balanced resuscitation is indicated. Aggressive administration of IV fluid may elevate the patient's blood pressure to levels that will disrupt any clot that has formed and result in recurrence of bleeding that had ceased because of blood clotting and hypotension. Prehospital care practitioners must achieve a delicate balance: maintain a blood pressure that provides perfusion to vital organs without restoring blood pressure to elevated or even normal ranges, which may reinitiate bleeding sites in the abdomen or pelvis. In the absence of TBI, the target systolic blood pressure is 80 to 90 mm Hg (mean arterial pressure of 60 to 65 mm Hg).

REFERENCES AND FURTHER READING

Irving T, Menon R, Ciantar E. Trauma during pregnancy. *BJA Educ.* 2021;21(1):10-19. doi:10.1016/j.bjae.2020.08.005

National Association of Emergency Medical Technicians. *PHTLS: Prehospital Trauma Life Support.* 10th ed. Burlington, MA: Public Safety Group; 2023.

Ng WM, Lee WF, Cheah SO, Chung YEL, Lee CY, Lim BL. Peri-mortem caesarean section after traumatic arrest: Crisis resource management. *Am J Emerg Med.* 2018;36(12):2338.e1-2338.e3. doi:10.1016/j.ajem.2018.08.078

Schwerin DL, Mohney S. EMS pain assessment and management. In: *StatPearls* [Internet]. StatPearls Publishing. Updated May 8, 2022. Accessed May 13, 2022. https://www.ncbi.nlm.nih.gov/books/NBK554543/

Solano JJ, Clayton LM, Parks DJ, et al. Prehospital ketamine administration for excited delirium with illicit substance co-ingestion and subsequent intubation in the emergency department. *Prehospital Disaster Med.* 2021;36(6):697-701. doi:10.1017/s1049023x21000935.

Index

Note: Page numbers followed by *f* or *t* indicate material in figures or tables, respectively

intubation using sedatives/narcotics, 65, 65*f*
ischemia, 77
   organ tolerance, 78, 78*t*

J

JumpSTART (pediatric algorithm), 32
junctional hemorrhage, defined, 31

K

ketamine, 158, 158*f*
kyphosis, 129, 129*f*

L

lactic acid, 78, 79
laryngeal mask airway, 47, 48*f*
laryngeal tube airway (LTA), 47
larynx, 39
lifting nonambulatory injured
    patients, 140
lower airway, 39, 41
LTA. *See* laryngeal tube airway

M

mangled extremity, 171, 171*f*
MAP. *See* mean arterial pressure
MARCH (Massive bleeding, Airway,
    Respirations, Circulation, Head
    injury/Hypothermia) approach, 5
MASS (Move, Assess, Sort, Send) triage
    method, 32
mass-casualty incident (MCI), 32
mass-casualty triage, 32–35, 33*f*
  SALT triage algorithm, 32–35, 35*f*
  START triage algorithm, 32, 34*f*
mass effect/herniation, 108–109
MCI. *See* mass-casualty incident
McSwain, Norman E., 6
mean arterial pressure (MAP), 107, 108
mechanism of injury (MOI), 15
MOI. *See* mechanism of injury
morphine, 158
motor vehicle collisions (MVCs), 2, 14*f*
motor vehicle crashes, 106
motor vehicle incidents, 14*f*
muscular system, 166
musculoskeletal trauma
   assessment, 166–167, 167*f*
   management
     amputations, 171–172, 171f
     compartment syndrome, 169–171
     crush syndrome, 172
     dislocation, 169
     femur fracture, 169
     fractures, 167–168, 167–168f
     mangled extremity, 171, 171f

   pelvic fracture, 168–169
   pulseless extremities, 168, 169f
MVCs. *See* motor vehicle collisions

N

NAEMT. *See* National Association of
    Emergency Medical Technicians
nasopharyngeal airway (NPA), 47, 47*f*
nasopharynx, 39
National Association of Emergency
    Medical Technicians (NAEMT), 6
National Guidelines for Field Triage of
    Injured Patients, 21, 22*f*
National Safety Council (NSC), 3
neurologic examination, 122
nonaccidental burns, 143–144, 144*f*
nonpharmacologic pain management,
    155–156, 156–157*f*, 157*t*
normal end-tidal waveform, 69, 69*f*
NPA. *See* nasopharyngeal airway
NSC. *See* National Safety Council

O

obesity, 140
obstetric patient, 128
   hemorrhage care, 32
   spinal motion restriction in, 128, 128*f*
obstetric trauma
   management of, 164–165, 164*f*
   physical examination, 163–164, 163*f*
on-scene information-gathering process, 13
OPA. *See* oropharyngeal airway
open pneumothorax, 61, 61*f*
oropharyngeal airway (OPA), 47, 47*f*
oropharynx, 39
over-triaging, 21
oxygenation process, 58–59
   effects of trauma, 59

P

pain management
   nonpharmacologic pain management,
     155–156, 156–157*f*, 157*t*
   pharmacologic pain management,
     156–158, 157*f*
     fentanyl, 158, 158*f*
     ketamine, 158, 158*f*
     morphine, 158
   subjective *versus* objective, 155
Parkland formula, 149–150
partial-thickness burns, 142, 142*f*
PEA. *See* pulseless electrical activity
pediatric pain scale, 156
pediatric patients, 129–130, 130*f*
   airway management, 49–52, 50*f*
   assessment considerations, 25
   blood loss, 84

   hemorrhage care, 32
   sniffing position, 50, 50*f*
   spinal motion restriction in, 129–130,
     130*f*
pelvic fracture, 168–169
penetrating brain injury, 104–105
penetrating injuries, 60, 123, 159–160
periorbital ecchymosis, 105
pharmacologic pain management,
    156–158, 157*f*
   fentanyl, 158, 158*f*
   ketamine, 158, 158*f*
   morphine, 158
pharmacologically assisted intubation.
    See drug-assisted intubation
pharynx, 39
PHTLS. *See* Prehospital Trauma Life
    Support
pneumothorax
   open, 61, 61*f*
   tension, 62–63, 62*f*
post-event phase, trauma care, 8
pre-event phase, trauma care, 7–8
preferences
   defined, 6
   versus principles, 7
pregnant patient, 128, 128*f*
   assessment considerations, 25
   blood loss, 84
   spinal motion restriction in, 128, 128*f*
prehospital burn pitfalls, 143
Prehospital Trauma Life Support
    (PHTLS)
   assessment and treatment of trauma
     patients, 5–6
   communication and documentation, 9
   goals of, 3, 4*f*
   Golden Principles of, 155
   past, 6
   philosophy of, 4–5
   prepare for unpreventable, 8
   present, 6
   principles and preferences, 6–7
   team approach, 5, 5*f*
   trauma care, phases of, 7–9
   vision for future, 6
primary survey, 15–20, 160, 160*f*
   airway assessment, 43
   airway management, 16–18, 17*f*
   breathing, 18
   cervical spine stabilization, 16–18
   circulation, 18–19
   different populations, 16
   disability, 19–20
   expose/environment, 20, 20*f*
   exsanguinating hemorrhage, 16
   hemorrhage control, 28–32